Scientific Opportunities and Public Needs

Improving Priority Setting and Public Input at the National Institutes of Health

Committee on the NIH Research Priority-Setting Process

Health Sciences Policy Program

Health Sciences Section

INSTITUTE OF MEDICINE

IOM

NATIONAL ACADEMY PRESS
Washington, D.C. 1998

NATIONAL ACADEMY PRESS • 2101 Constitution Avenue, N.W. • Washington, D.C. 20418

NOTICE: The project that is the subject of this report was approved by the Governing Board of the National Research Council, whose members are drawn from the councils of the National Academy of Sciences, the National Academy of Engineering, and the Institute of Medicine. The members of the committee responsible for the report were chosen for their special competences and with regard for appropriate balance.

The Institute of Medicine was chartered in 1970 by the National Academy of Sciences to enlist distinguished members of the appropriate professions in the examination of policy matters pertaining to the health of the public. In this, the Institute acts under both the Academy's 1863 congressional charter responsibility to be an adviser to the federal government and its own initiative in identifying issues of medical care, research, and education. Dr. Kenneth I. Shine is president of the Institute of Medicine.

Support for this project was provided by funds from the National Institutes of Health (Contract No. N01-OD-4-2139). The views presented in this report are those of the Committee on the NIH Research Priority-Setting Process and are not necessarily those of the funding organization.

International Standard Book No. 0-309-06130-X

Additional copies of this report are available for sale from the National Academy Press, 2101 Constitution Avenue, N.W., Box 285, Washington, DC 20055. Call (800) 624-6242 or (202) 334-3313 (in the Washington metropolitan area), or visit the NAP's on-line bookstore at **http://www.nap.edu.**

The full text of this report is available on line at **http://www.nap.edu.**

For more information about the Institute of Medicine, visit the IOM home page at **http://www2. nas.edu/iom.**

Printed in the United States of America

The serpent has been a symbol of long life, healing, and knowledge among almost all cultures and religions since the beginning of recorded history. The image adopted as a logotype by the Institute of Medicine is based on a relief carving from ancient Greece, now held by the Staatliche Museen in Berlin.

First Printing, July 1998
Second Printing, September 1998

COMMITTEE ON THE NIH RESEARCH PRIORITY-SETTING PROCESS

LEON E. ROSENBERG*,† (*Chair*), Professor, Department of Molecular Biology, and Woodrow Wilson School of Public and International Affairs, Princeton University

JOHN ALDERETE, Professor, Department of Microbiology, University of Texas Health Science Center at San Antonio

KENNETH B. CHANCE, Dean and Professor of Endodontics, Meharry Medical College School of Dentistry

CARON CHESS, Director, Center for Environmental Communication, Cook College, Rutgers University

PURNELL CHOPPIN,*,† President, Howard Hughes Medical Institute

JAMES W. CURRAN,* Dean and Professor of Epidemiology, The Rollins School of Public Health, Emory University

DAVID CUTLER, Professor, Department of Economics, Littauer Center, Harvard University

SUE DONALDSON,* Professor and Dean, School of Nursing and Professor of Physiology, School of Medicine, Johns Hopkins University

BARUCH FISCHHOFF,* University Professor, Department of Engineering and Public Policy, Department of Social and Decision Sciences, Carnegie Mellon University

SID GILMAN,* William J. Herdman Professor and Chair, Department of Neurology, University of Michigan

ROBERT L. HILL,*,† James B. Duke Professor, Department of Biochemistry, Duke University Medical Center

RALPH HORWITZ,* Chair and Professor, Department of Internal Medicine, Yale University School of Medicine

THOMAS KELLY,† Boury Professor and Chairman, Department of Molecular Biology and Genetics, Johns Hopkins University

ANNE PETERSEN, Senior Vice President, Programs, W.K. Kellogg Foundation

SUSAN C. SCRIMSHAW,* Dean and Professor of Community Health Sciences, School of Public Health, University of Illinois at Chicago

ROGER UNGER,† Professor of Internal Medicine, Center for Diabetes Research, University of Texas Southwestern Medical Center

MYRL WEINBERG, President, National Health Council

LINDA S. WILSON,* President, Radcliffe College

ADAM YARMOLINSKY,* Regents Professor of Public Policy in the University of Maryland System

---

*Member of the Institute of Medicine.

†Member of the National Academy of Sciences.

Committee Liaisons

HARVEY R. COLTEN,* Dean and Vice President for Medical Affairs, Northwestern University School of Medicine
JOSEPH T. COYLE,* Eben S. Draper Professor of Psychiatry and Neuroscience Chair, Consolidated Department of Psychiatry, Harvard Medical School
JOHN D. STOBO,* President, University of Texas Medical Branch

Study Staff

ANDREW POPE, Director, Health Sciences Policy Program
GEOFFREY FRENCH, Research Associate

Consultants

KATHI HANNA
MICHAEL McGEARY

Copy Editor

MICHAEL HAYES

Section Staff

CHARLES H. EVANS, JR., Head, Health Sciences Section
ROBERT COOK-DEEGAN, Director, National Cancer Policy Board
LINDA DEPUGH, Administrative Assistant
JAMAINE TINKER, Financial Associate

---

*Member of the Institute of Medicine.

REVIEWERS

This report has been reviewed in draft form by individuals chosen for their diverse perspectives and technical expertise, in accordance with procedures approved by the National Research Council's Report Review Committee. The purpose of this independent review is to provide candid and critical comments that will assist the Institute of Medicine in making the published report as sound as possible and to ensure that the report meets institutional standards for objectivity, evidence, and responsiveness to the study charge. The content of the final report is the responsibility of the Institute of Medicine and the study committee and not the responsibility of the reviewers. The review comments and draft manuscript remain confidential to protect the integrity of the deliberative process. The committee wishes to thank the following individuals, who are neither officials nor employees of the Institute of Medicine, for their participation in the review of this report:

JOHN ABELSON,† California Institute of Technology
DONALD D. BROWN,† Carnegie Institution of Washington
MICHAEL S. BROWN,*,† University of Texas Southwestern Medical Center
JAMES EBERT,*,† Marine Biological Laboratory, Woods Hole
ROBIN ELLIOTT, Parkinson's Disease Foundation
HARMON J. EYRE, American Cancer Society
MARC W. KIRSCHNER,† Harvard Medical School
S. ROBERT LEVINE, Juvenile Diabetes Foundation International
ROBERT LEVY,* American Home Products Corp.
MARSHALL LICHTMAN, Leukemia Society of America
DOROTHY RICE,* University of California, San Francisco
PAUL ROGERS,* Hogan & Hartson
CHARLES SANDERS,* Glaxo, Inc.
HOWARD K. SCHACHMAN,† University of California, Berkeley
MORTON N. SWARTZ,* Massachusetts General Hospital
SAMUEL THIER,* Partners Health Care System, Inc.
LOWELL WEICKER, University of Virginia
MYRON WEISFELDT,* Columbia University and past president, American Heart Association

While the individuals listed above have provided many constructive comments and suggestions, responsibility for the final content of this report rests solely with the authoring committee and the Institute of Medicine.

---

*Member of the Institute of Medicine.

†Member of the National Academy of Sciences.

Preface

The United States is preeminent in medical research. Since World War II this country has fashioned a medical research system—with government, academia, and industry at its core—that is a source of great national pride and the envy of the world. The federal government is the single largest sponsor of this research, committing more than $16 billion of public funds in the current fiscal year (1998). Of this total, the vast majority—$13.6 billion—is appropriated to the National Institutes of Health (NIH). Given the size of this public investment and the likelihood that it will be increased significantly in the immediate future and given the mission of NIH—"to uncover new knowledge that will lead to better health for everyone"—it should come as no surprise that there is intense interest in how NIH sets its priorities, that is, how it allocates its sizable budget. How could it be otherwise? Every one of us wants to live a long and healthy life. Every sick person—woman, man, or child—wants researchers to find new ways to make him or her well or to improve the quality of life for those who are disabled, regardless of whether the ailment is common or rare, acute or chronic, life-threatening or self-limiting.

We must acknowledge that setting priorities at NIH is an awesome task. Not only must the leadership of NIH answer to the executive branch and to the U.S. Congress, it must work with all of its constituencies—scientists, health care providers, patients, voluntary health groups and patient advocates, and industry executives—before making its fateful decisions. The quality and quantity of excellent science that it has supported, the widespread respect for it in and out of government, and its favored position in the annual congressional appropriations process signify that, over time, NIH must be doing many things right. Yet, we must also acknowledge that the recent request from Congress that the Institute of Medicine conduct an independent assessment of research priority setting at NIH and that the evaluation be completed within 6 months signifies, just as clearly, that there is at least a perception that some things are not right. It is apparent that some segments of the public, in general, and its representatives in Congress, in particular, are dissatisfied enough to ask for ways to improve the current process.

This committee was charged with examining four issues related to setting priorities at NIH: allocation criteria, the decision-making process, mechanisms for public input, and the impact of congressional directives. Despite the nearly impossible constraints imposed by the study's time line, we took this broad charge seriously. To grasp the approach that NIH currently uses, we heard in person from the director of NIH, most of the institute directors, and many of the directors of offices housed within the director's office. To understand the tensions surrounding public input, we held a full-day public meeting at which we received verbal and written testimony from patients, advocacy and interest groups, foundations, and professional societies. To understand Congress's rationale for requesting the study, we interviewed legislative aides from key offices. To expand our collective knowledge base, we reviewed many current and past publications relevant to our charge.

As we listened and deliberated, several things became clear to me. First, the country has extraordinarily high expectations of NIH. To some, NIH has become a virtual surrogate for the U.S. Department of Health and Human Services, being encouraged to expand its purview well beyond research. We heard from no one who wants to dismantle NIH; we heard from many who wanted their "cause" to be embraced by NIH; we heard from all that NIH must excel at everything it does because what it does is so important to the hopes and aspirations of people everywhere.

Second, there is a sense that NIH has evolved mechanisms for judging scientific opportunity and merit that surpass its capabilities for assessing and being influenced by public health needs. Estimating research spending by disease and developing metrics for spending according to disease burden (e.g., incidence, mortality, disability, and cost) must be done more systematically and more thoroughly than they are currently done because not doing so leads some to conclude, incorrectly I believe, that NIH cares more about curiosity than cure, more about fundamental science than clinical application.

Third, there is frustration on the part of some groups about not being listened to and heard by NIH. We heard repeatedly that some institutes, and particularly the Office of the Director, lack mechanisms for orderly, regular public input and outreach. As the authority of the director over priority setting has increased, the demand to influence that office has become louder.

Fourth, there is a lack of understanding about how NIH priority setting "works." NIH has not crafted simple communications that make its priority-setting processes as transparent as possible to its many publics. NIH has not developed sufficient communications tools to satisfy people that allocation decisions are made on the basis of equity and justice, as well as scientific opportunity.

Each of these observations has been converted to recommendations that reflect the committee's consensus. Our recommendations address each of the committee's charges, but there is a single theme that runs through them. It is that NIH must revamp its approach to public input and outreach—at every level—without delay. This will strengthen the priority-setting process in many ways. It will underscore that openness is as important to the process as such other valued qualities as expertise, innovation, and objectivity. It will provide NIH leaders more ways to demonstrate that they share the public's view that NIH exists to improve health through research. It will enhance the public's understanding of the complexities of decision making at NIH. Finally, it will give Congress additional confidence that it can delegate priority setting to NIH leadership knowing that a broader range of views will be sought and welcomed before decisions are made.

I would like to thank the many people who have made it possible for this report to be completed on schedule: first and foremost, the members of the committee who met and overcame the many challenges of our difficult task with a commendable blend of experience, energy, collegiality, and wisdom; second, the staff of the Institute of Medicine, without whom we would have foundered; third, the leadership of NIH, who educated us about this agency; and fourth, and perhaps most important, the public, who reminded us of the purpose of NIH and of the democratic ideals that must permeate effective stewardship of a federal agency.

Leon E. Rosenberg, M.D.
Chair

Acronyms

ACD	Advisory Committee to the Director
DHHS	U.S. Department of Health and Human Services
FIC	John E. Fogarty International Center
FY	fiscal year
IOM	Institute of Medicine
NCI	National Cancer Institute, NIH
NCRR	National Center for Research Resources, NIH
NEI	National Eye Institute, NIH
NHGRI	National Human Genome Research Institute, NIH
NHLBI	National Heart, Lung, and Blood Institute, NIH
NIA	National Institute on Aging, NIH
NIAAA	National Institute on Alcohol Abuse and Alcoholism, NIH
NIAID	National Institute of Allergy and Infectious Diseases, NIH
NIAMS	National Institute of Arthritis and Musculoskeletal and Skin Diseases, NIH
NICHD	National Institute of Child Health and Human Development, NIH
NIDA	National Institute on Drug Abuse, NIH

NIDCD	National Institute on Deafness and Other Communication Disorders, NIH
NIDDK	National Institute of Diabetes and Digestive and Kidney Diseases, NIH
NIDR	National Institute of Dental Research, NIH
NIEHS	National Institute of Environmental Health Sciences, NIH
NIGMS	National Institute of General Medical Sciences, NIH
NIH	National Institutes of Health
NIMH	National Institute of Mental Health, NIH
NINDS	National Institute of Neurological Disorders and Stroke, NIH
NINR	National Institute of Nursing Research, NIH
NLM	National Library of Medicine, NIH
NSF	National Science Foundation
OMB	Office of Management and Budget
PHS	Public Health Service
R&D	research and development
RFA	request for application
RPG	research project grant

Contents

Scientific Opportunities and Public Needs

Executive Summary

The National Institutes of Health (NIH) is the leading federal agency supporting research related to improving the nation's health. The scientists and clinicians whom it has helped train and support have consistently been at the forefront of research discoveries that have advanced fundamental knowledge of human biology and of better ways to treat or prevent disease and promote good health. Over the past 50 years, NIH as an institution has played a major role in the explosion of knowledge that has amounted to a revolution in biology.

NIH's success has earned it steadily increasing budgets even when the overall federal budget has been tight, as it has been in recent years. Although the NIH budget for the current fiscal year (1998) is more than $13 billion and both the administration and the U.S. Congress have promised a substantial increase for 1999, it will never be large enough to meet every need or fund every promising lead. Choices must be made and priorities must be set.

Concerns about priority setting in the allocation of NIH research funding come from several sources. First, some members of Congress believe that there should be more of a correlation between the allocation of funding by disease and the distribution of disease burdens and costs in the population. Second, more and more disease-specific interest groups have begun campaigning for increases in NIH funding related to particular diseases. Additionally, many of these groups do not feel that NIH listens or responds to their inputs. Finally, the leadership of the health committees in Congress has become increasingly uncomfortable with intervening in research priority setting at NIH, for example, by mandating specific funding set-asides, new programs or institutions focused on specific diseases, or the use of particular research mechanisms or by trying to push research advances in specific areas in other ways. For these reasons, this committee has been asked to evaluate the processes for setting priorities at NIH, particularly NIH's mechanisms for obtaining public input and the role of Congress in directing the allocation of funding among areas of research.

In setting priorities, NIH must also adapt to a changing policy environment. Despite having a growing budget, scientific research opportunities have grown even more rapidly, as has awareness of health problems as the population ages and as globalization exposes the U.S. population to emerging or reemerging infectious diseases.

To meet the expectations of the American people and fulfill the agency's mission, NIH's leaders must pursue many objectives. Two of the most important are (1) to identify the public's health needs, reducing the burdens of illness by developing better methods of prevention, diagnosis, treatment, and rehabilitation, and (2) to extend the basic knowledge base to lead to even better methods in the future. These two objectives are complementary and must be pursued with equal intensities if NIH is going to be successful. A third important objective is to communicate to the public and health providers the current state of scientific knowledge and the implications of research advances for improving the nation's health. Box 1 describes some of NIH's constituencies.

BOX 1 NIH Constituencies

NIH interacts with various external constituencies who have a stake in research priority setting. These include:

- research scientists in universities, colleges, medical centers, and other research institutions outside NIH who conduct most of the research funded by NIH;
- clinicians who apply research results and who can help identify research needs (physicians, including specialized physicians, nurses, dentists, pharmacists, social workers, psychologists, public health practitioners, and other allied health practitioners);
- organized voluntary groups and individuals active in advocating for those with specific diseases or medical conditions;
- organizations and individuals who represent population groups with special health problems (members of particular ethnic groups, low-income populations, women, elderly people, children, etc.);
- Congress, which provides NIH with the authority and funding to carry out its mission, which oversees its effectiveness, and with which NIH must maintain good communication about priorities; and
- media who communicate research results and NIH activities and who thus play an important role in helping the public understand the research enterprise.

Identifying the burden of illness, however, is not a straightforward task. As indicated in the NIH booklet "Setting Research Priorities at the National Institutes of Health" (National Institutes of Health, 1997b) (referred to hereafter as Setting Research Priorities), there are many ways to measure the burden of disease because the problem can be analyzed and interpreted from many different perspectives. These are all relevant because the concept of the burden of disease is very broad.

> When applied to illness, the burden includes the heavy load borne by society in providing services to prevent, cure, and care for the sick. It also includes the substantial losses of output to the economy due to disease, disability, and death. The burden on the family in caring for and accommodating a sick member of the household can also be severe. Finally, there is the burden of pain, discomfort, and suffering of each sick person and that of anguish and grief of relatives and friends (Institute of Medicine, 1976:2).

Assessing the burden of disease takes into account the fact that the benefits of past research have not reached everyone, indicated by significant differentials in disease rates and outcomes among different socioeconomic and ethnic groups. Also, about half the nation's health care costs result from unhealthy behaviors and environments, which pose major research challenges. In addition, state-of-the-art screening, diagnostic procedures, and treatments are not reaching everyone, resulting in unnecessary burdens of undetected or poorly treated diseases, and patient and provider knowledge could be improved through education. All of these factors must be weighed and balanced in the priority-setting process.

The committee assessed NIH's priority-setting process in light of the agency's mission and objectives and the changing policy environment. Are the criteria adequate? Is the process for implementing them working? Given the objective of responding to health needs as well as scientific opportunity, in conjunction with the expansion of organized disease-specific interest groups, are the mechanisms for public input adequate, or can they be changed to increase the complementarity between NIH's goals of responding to health needs and scientific opportunity? Can Congress, the holder of the public purse strings, be assured that NIH has a rigorous process for priority setting in which the full range of considerations is taken into account in planning programs and allocating funding?

The committee concludes that NIH's system for setting priorities has generally served NIH and the nation well in supporting research to improve human health, but some changes would strengthen it, especially in mechanisms for exchanging information and concerns with interested individuals and groups. The process by which NIH sets its research priorities should more fully engage the public (i.e., the public should have greater opportunity to learn about and provide input into the priority-setting process) in a process that is led by the director, guided by reasonable criteria, and well informed by robust analyses of health statistics. The process should be open and understandable, include multiyear strategic planning, and give appropriate consideration to the competing needs of scientific opportunity and disease burden. Effective implementation of such a process would improve public access to the process and limit the need for congressional directives.

CRITERIA FOR PRIORITY SETTING

The committee reviewed the major criteria that NIH uses in its overall priority setting. These criteria were explicitly laid out in Setting Research Priorities, and the committee concluded that they are generally reasonable and useful both for allocating research resources and for enabling organized interest groups, members of Congress, and members of the public to understand and evaluate NIH's program. The criteria are

- public health needs,
- scientific quality of the research,
- potential for scientific progress (the existence of promising pathways and qualified investigators),
- portfolio diversification along the broad and expanding frontiers of research, and
- adequate support of infrastructure (human capital, equipment and instrumentation, and facilities).

The committee wants to be sure, however, that the conceptualization of the first criterion, public health needs, be broadened beyond the medical model implied in the discussion of the criterion in the booklet to include the preservation and maintenance of health and function.

> ***Recommendation 1.*** **The committee generally supports the criteria that NIH uses for priority setting and recommends that NIH continue to use these criteria in a balanced way to cover the full spectrum of research related to human health.**

To enhance the legitimacy of and support for its priority-setting and resource allocation processes, NIH should work to increase the level of understanding of its criteria by the general public and of how they are implemented and should engage in regular evaluations of how the criteria are used and of their impacts. The Setting Research Priorities booklet and other documents are not as effective at gaining public understanding as they could be, for example, in informing citizens who are concerned about health and particular diseases about how they can become involved (an issue addressed more fully below in the section Mechanisms for Public Input).

Recommendation 2. **NIH should make clear its mechanisms for implementing its criteria for setting priorities and should evaluate their use and effectiveness.**

The committee found that some of the information needed for priority setting, especially data on disease burden and costs, is obtained rather informally and concluded that NIH should be more systematic in obtaining and analyzing such data. It should be kept in mind, however, that there is no simple metric for the use of these data, and the relationship between such data and allocations of research funding will not be simple because health problems are not equally ripe for research advances.

Recommendation 3. **In setting priorities, NIH should strengthen its analysis and use of health data, such as burdens and costs of diseases, and of data on the impact of research on the health of the public.**

Individuals and groups concerned about specific health problems or health research often use NIH-generated data on spending by specific disease or area of research to assess the overall research portfolio. The data are not of the quality that they could be, however, and NIH should work to improve the data and to better explain the data to the public. Calculations of spending by disease should include not only all research directly related to the disease but also research projects on fundamental areas indirectly related to that disease. Users of the data should know that such calculations reflect the best estimates of all NIH spending in particular areas and that fundamental science is essential to understanding the etiology and progression of disease.

NIH should also collect and analyze data on health research spending by others, such as other federal agencies, industry, nonprofit health organizations that fund research, foundations, or other countries. This should help identify gaps, overlaps, and opportunities for joint efforts and ensure that NIH invests wisely in areas and approaches that no one else is funding, provides the appropriate coordination, and supports the training of personnel and the other infrastructure needed in the national research enterprise.

Recommendation 4. **NIH should improve the quality and analysis of its data on funding by disease and should include both direct and related expenditures.**

PRIORITY-SETTING PROCESSES

Priority setting is decentralized at NIH, which is appropriate for a research organization in which those closest to a problem are in the best position to decide on approaches and in which expertise is highly specialized. The priority-setting processes also vary from institute to institute and from area to area within institutes. Some such variation is appropriate, because the institutes vary in their missions, histories, leadership, sizes, and complexities. The committee did find that some institutes and programs have priority-setting processes that incorporate a broader range of inputs and views, including those of nonresearchers and nonclinicians.

More recently, NIH has been making decisions on priorities and funding allocations that are more centralized than in the past; that is, NIH is looking across traditionally independent institutes and centers and focusing on certain crosscutting needs and opportunities where joint or unified action is desirable. This trend stems from the growing realization that common biological processes underlie diseases that were previously seen as different or that important diseases and other health problems are more complex than was previously thought, affect more organs and processes than was previously realized, and happen to be addressed in more than one institute.

The committee concluded that the Office of the Director of NIH needs an increased capacity to analyze such crosscutting needs and opportunities and to interact with the public (the latter process-related issue is addressed separately below). Improvement requires a more central role for the NIH director and more uniformity in the data and analyses presented to the Office of the Director.

> ***Recommendation 5.*** **In exercising the overall authority to oversee and coordinate the priority-setting process, the NIH director should receive from the directors of all of the institutes and centers multiyear strategic plans, including budget scenarios, in a standard format on an annual basis.**

In any organization, change toward centralization raises concerns about accountability. As the authority of the director is strengthened, greater accountability of the director's office could be achieved through a strengthened Advisory Committee to the Director, one that is more actively engaged in the NIH priority-setting process and that has a broader base of membership, especially among its public members.

> ***Recommendation 6.*** **The director of NIH should increase the involvement of the Advisory Committee to the Director in the priority-setting process. The diversity of the committee's membership should be increased, particularly with respect to its public members.**

MECHANISMS FOR PUBLIC INPUT

Although a major criterion in research priority setting is public health needs, the committee found that NIH's interaction with various kinds of publics is generally weak compared with NIH's interaction with the research community. This is especially true for the Office of the Director of NIH, which does not have adequate channels through which members of the public can express their concerns to NIH or through which they can receive information about the broad scope of effort being made in the fields with which they are concerned.

This structural weakness has important implications: first, because patient advocacy groups have become better organized and more proactive on behalf of their interests and have greatly increased their appeals to Congress to intervene to adjust NIH research priorities; second, because congressional leaders have expressed a strong desire to avoid mandates and earmarks in favor of particular diseases and to let NIH set research priorities; and third, because the NIH director has increased his role in priority setting (partly by exercising additional authorities granted to him by Congress). This confluence of events highlights the need for improved communication between the public and NIH.

NIH should engage the public to a greater extent in informing the process by which NIH sets its research priorities. The following three recommendations are intended to provide the public with more opportunities to present their views regarding research needs and to receive information about research and the priority-setting process at NIH.

> ***Recommendation* 7. NIH should establish an Office of Public Liaison in the Office of the Director and, where offices performing such a function are not already in place, in each institute. These offices should document, in a standard format, their public outreach, input, and response mechanisms. The director's Office of Public Liaison should review and evaluate these mechanisms and identify best practices.**

The Offices of Public Liaison are meant to serve several purposes: (1) they provide an easily identifiable point of contact for individuals and groups who have an interest or concern; (2) they are a place where members of Congress can refer constituents who want to obtain information or to raise concerns; and (3) they conduct an active program of outreach to and interaction with constituency groups. The NIH director's Office of Public Liaison will oversee and coordinate the institutes' Offices of Public Liaison, serve as a point of contact for individuals or groups who are dealing with crosscutting issues or who do not have a specific institute to contact, and staff the Director's Council of Public Representatives (discussed below).

***Recommendation 8.* The director of NIH should establish and appropriately staff a Director's Council of Public Representatives, chaired by the NIH director, to facilitate interactions between NIH and the general public.**

The Director's Council of Public Representatives—an advisory group made up of citizens who are either patients, family members of patients, or advocates for patients—serves to elevate public input into the priority-setting process to the highest level of NIH in a systematic and periodic manner. Importantly, the Council will not set priorities regarding the NIH budget or its research programs. That is, it is not intended to serve as a forum for advocacy groups to lobby the NIH director for research dollars. Rather, it is intended to serve as a mechanism for NIH to receive valuable and thoughtful perspectives on its research programs from those who are in some way affected by disease and disability and who are therefore advocates for a healthy NIH and for NIH to provide information about its research and priority-setting process as part of a two-way exchange of information.

Together with the Offices of Public Liaison, the Director's Council of Public Representatives would permit continual interaction between NIH and the public. The Council would allow the NIH director to hear periodically from representatives of a spectrum of interest groups; the Offices of Public Liaison, which would be staff offices that function on a daily basis, unlike the Council, would provide information to and receive input from interested groups and congressional offices and would staff the Council in the Office of the Director. Figure 1 shows the proposed placement of the Offices of Public Liaison and the Director's Council of Public Representatives within the current organization at NIH.

***Recommendation 9.* The public membership of NIH policy and program advisory groups should be selected to represent a broad range of public constituencies.**

NIH has long-standing mechanisms by which to include public or lay members on top-level advisory bodies. In the institutes, these councils provide advice and guidance on their research programs and funding decisions by providing the second layer of review (the first being peer review through the study sections). Thus, public representatives play a role in the priority-setting process and provide advice on funding decisions. NIH also reserves slots for public members on the Advisory Committee to the Director. It does not appear, however, that advocates for patients or special populations are regularly considered for these advisory committee memberships, despite numerous examples of cases in which such arrangements have been constructive and positive. Not using this mechanism to receive public input is a missed opportunity and has resulted in the perception of some groups that NIH does not encourage public input at the highest levels of its advisory processes.

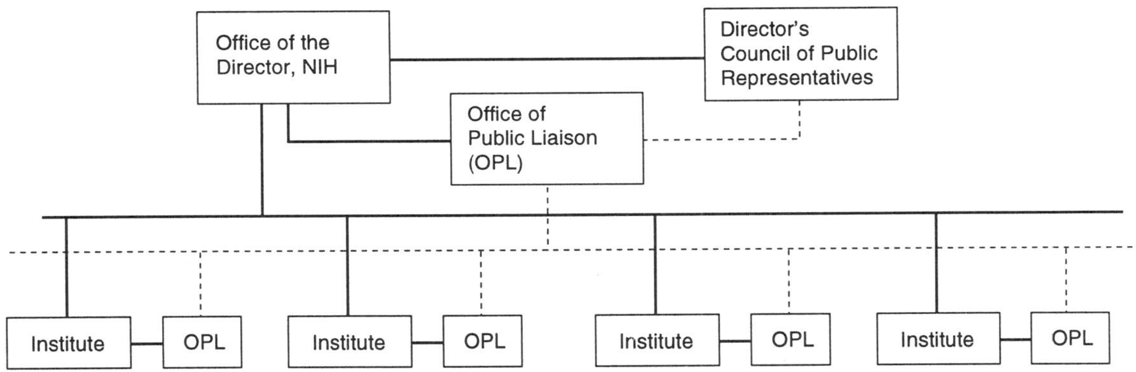

FIGURE 1 Proposed placement of the Offices of Public Liaison and the Director's Council of Public Representatives within the current organization at NIH.

These recommendations are not intended to replace the existing criteria for priority setting. They are intended to enhance and reinforce existing NIH mechanisms through which the voices of the public can be heard in a constructive and open manner. The committee believes that public input, which has been important in sustaining the growth and stature of NIH, is an important component of the priority-setting process and, if used wisely by NIH when setting research priorities, will make for a stronger and more responsive NIH. It also believes that although implementation of these recommendations will not supersede or remove the potential for appeals to Congress, their enactment will reduce the need for such appeals.

The new organizational mechanisms proposed to improve public input have the potential to increase, in the short term, organizational costs and complexity. In the long run, however, the committee believes that the contribution made by these offices and the Council will prove to be cost-effective in terms of carrying out NIH's mission to improve health through research and will contribute to overall goodwill on the part of the public and Congress toward NIH.

CONGRESSIONAL ROLE

Congress has always taken a special interest in NIH and has usually provided for larger budgets than administrations request. Congress has also often directed NIH in fairly specific ways, requiring the establishment of research programs, setting aside specific amounts of funding for research on designated problems, mandating the creation of research centers, institutes, or other specific mechanisms, and so forth.

Congress has the authority and the responsibility to intervene if it thinks that NIH is neglecting an opportunity or is not responsive to a need. Members of Congress recognize that it would be better for NIH to make the detailed decisions on how to approach problems.

The committee believes that if NIH revises its priority-setting system in the ways recommended above, Congress will be more likely to grant NIH (which, it is hoped, will be informed by stronger public input) the primary role in setting its research priorities. The text of the report includes some guidelines first offered by an Institute of Medicine committee in 1984 for Congress to use in deciding whether to mandate major organizational changes.

> ***Recommendation 10.*** **The U.S. Congress should use its authority to mandate specific research programs, establish levels of funding for them, and implement new organizational entities only when other approaches have proven inadequate. NIH should provide Congress with analyses of how NIH is responding to requests for such major changes and whether these requests can be addressed within existing mechanisms.**

If NIH is to have more autonomy in organizing and managing its research programs, it is incumbent on the agency to engage in periodic reviews of its organizational structure and planning and budgeting systems and to explain the results to Congress and the public.

> ***Recommendation 11.* The director of NIH should periodically review and report on the organizational structure of NIH, in light of changes in science and the health needs of the public.**

The committee questions whether NIH, especially the Office of the Director, has adequate resources to operate an effective priority-setting system. Providing the Office of the Director of NIH with adequate resources for analysis and interface with the public would make research priority setting more effective.

> ***Recommendation 12.* Congress should adjust the levels of funding for research management and support so that NIH can implement improvements in the priority-setting process, including stronger analytical, planning, and public interface capacities.**

BOX 2 The Committee's Recommendations

Criteria for Priority Setting

Recommendation 1. The committee generally supports the criteria that NIH uses for priority setting and recommends that NIH continue to use these criteria in a balanced way to cover the full spectrum of research related to human health.

Recommendation 2. NIH should make clear its mechanisms for implementing its criteria for setting priorities and should evaluate their use and effectiveness.

Recommendation 3. In setting priorities, NIH should strengthen its analysis and use of health data, such as burdens and costs of diseases, and of data on the impact of research on the health of the public.

Recommendation 4. NIH should improve the quality and analysis of its data on funding by disease and should include both direct and related expenditures.

Priority-Setting Processes

Recommendation 5. In exercising the overall authority to oversee and coordinate the priority-setting process, the NIH director should receive from the directors of all of the institutes and centers multiyear strategic plans, including budget scenarios, in a standard format on an annual basis.

Continued

BOX 2 *Continued*

Recommendation 6. The director of NIH should increase the involvement of the Advisory Committee to the Director in the priority-setting process. The diversity of the committee's membership should be increased, particularly with respect to its public members.

Mechanisms for Public Input

NIH should engage the public to a greater extent in informing the process by which NIH sets its research priorities, as illustrated by the following:

Recommendation 7. NIH should establish an Office of Public Liaison in the Office of the Director and, where offices performing such a function are not already in place, in each institute. These offices should document, in a standard format, their public outreach, input, and response mechanisms. The director's Office of Public Liaison should review and evaluate these mechanisms and identify best practices.

Recommendation 8. The director of NIH should establish and appropriately staff a Director's Council of Public Representatives, chaired by the NIH director, to facilitate interactions between NIH and the general public.

Recommendation 9. The public membership of NIH policy and program advisory groups should be selected to represent a broad range of public constituencies.

Congressional Action

Recommendation 10. The U.S. Congress should use its authority to mandate specific research programs, establish levels of funding for them, and implement new organizational entities only when other approaches have proven inadequate. NIH should provide Congress with analyses of how NIH is responding to requests for such major changes and whether these requests can be addressed within existing mechanisms.

Recommendation 11. The director of NIH should periodically review and report on the organizational structure of NIH, in light of changes in science and the health needs of the public.

Recommendation 12. Congress should adjust the levels of funding for research management and support so that NIH can implement improvements in the priority-setting process, including stronger analytical, planning, and public interface capacities.

1

Introduction

The Institute of Medicine (IOM) was asked by the National Institutes of Health (NIH) "to conduct a comprehensive study of the policies and processes used by NIH to determine funding allocations for biomedical research" in accordance with a congressional provision (U.S. Congress, 1997a). The U.S. House and U.S. Senate authorization and appropriations committees requested that IOM present findings, conclusions, and recommendations "for improvements in the NIH research funding policies and processes and for any necessary congressional action." Specifically, the congressional committees asked that IOM "assess:

- the factors or criteria used by NIH to determine funding allocations for disease research,
- the process by which research funding decisions are made,
- the mechanisms for public input into the priority-setting process, and
- the impact of statutory directives on research funding decisions."

IOM was asked to conduct the study and submit a report in time to inform congressional consideration of reauthorization legislation in 1998 as well as of fiscal year (FY) 1999 appropriations (that is, during the second session of the 105th Congress). To comply with this request, IOM agreed to deliver the report by July 1, 1998, 5 months after the study began. The committee process is described below, after the following review of the background of issues concerning research priority setting at NIH.

BACKGROUND

NIH is located in the U.S. Department of Health and Human Services (DHHS) with other health-related agencies of the federal government, including the Agency for Health Care Policy and Research, Centers for Disease Control and Prevention, Food and Drug Administration, Health Care Financing Administration, and Health Resources and Services Administration. NIH is the primary agency for research on health, accounting for 94 percent of DHHS's budget for health research and development (calculated from data from the National Science Foundation [NSF; 1997a:Table 8]).

NIH, which traces its roots to 1887, has grown steadily in size and scope, especially since the end of World War II, when the National Cancer Institute (NCI) was the only separately organized entity and the budget was $3 million. Currently, in FY 1998, there are 21 institutes and centers addressing different aspects of health research and several other major organizational units, and the budget for all NIH institutes and centers (see Box 1-1) is $13.6 billion.

BOX 1-1 Institutes and Centers of the National Institutes of Health

John E. Fogarty International Center
National Cancer Institute
National Center for Research Resources
National Eye Institute
National Heart, Lung, and Blood Institute
National Human Genome Research Institute
National Institute of Allergy and Infectious Diseases
National Institute of Arthritis and Musculoskeletal and Skin Diseases
National Institute of Child Health and Human Development
National Institute of Dental Research
National Institute of Diabetes and Digestive and Kidney Diseases
National Institute of Environmental Health Sciences
National Institute of General Medical Sciences
National Institute of Mental Health
National Institute of Neurological Disorders and Stroke
National Institute of Nursing Research
National Institute on Aging
National Institute on Alcohol Abuse and Alcoholism
National Institute on Deafness and Other Communication Disorders
National Institute on Drug Abuse
National Library of Medicine

According to the *NIH Manual* (National Institutes of Health, 1994b), "The National Institutes of Health is the steward of biomedical and behavioral research for the nation. Its mission is science in pursuit of fundamental knowledge about the nature and behavior of living systems and the application of that knowledge to extend healthy life and reduce the burdens of illness and disability." As put more succinctly on its web page, the mission of NIH is "to uncover new knowledge that will lead to better health for everyone" (National Institutes of Health, 1998b).

NIH carries out its mission by supporting research of many kinds, funding the training of new researchers, and fostering communication of research results to health care professionals and the public. How it allocates its resources among and within these activities—that is, how it sets priorities—is of great importance to the public, the media, organized disease-specific interest groups, health care providers, and researchers themselves because of widespread and deeply held interest in the impact of NIH on health and disease and on the productivity of the nation's health research enterprise (see Box 1-2 for a list of NIH constituencies).

There are many ways to view the allocation of NIH's budget, reflecting its diverse portfolio of activities. Each cut or dimension emphasizes different aspects of NIH and priority setting.

BOX 1-2 NIH Constituencies

NIH interacts with various external constituencies who have a stake in research priority setting. These include:

- research scientists in universities, colleges, medical centers, and other research institutions outside NIH who conduct most of the research funded by NIH;
- clinicians who apply research results and who can help identify research needs (physicians, including specialized physicians, nurses, dentists, pharmacists, social workers, psychologists, public health practitioners, and other allied health practitioners);
- organized voluntary groups and individuals active in advocating for those with specific diseases or medical conditions;
- organizations and individuals who represent population groups with special health problems (members of particular ethnic groups, low-income populations, women, elderly people, children, etc.);
- Congress, which provides NIH with the authority and funding to carry out its mission, which oversees its effectiveness, and with which NIH must maintain good communication about priorities; and
- media (reporters, editors, and others) who communicate research results and NIH activities and who thus play an important role in helping the public understand the research enterprise.

Although NIH is the largest single funder of health research in the United States, it is part of a much larger research enterprise in which industry—such as pharmaceutical companies and biotechnology firms—spends more (about $19 billion and $8 billion, respectively) on research (Pharmaceutical Research and Manufacturers of America, 1997; Biotechnology Industry Organization, 1998). Within this larger system, NIH supports the basic research to gain fundamental knowledge about health and disease processes that the private sector will not support because it may not be profitable, while companies focus their research on applications, such as new drugs, diagnostic tools, and medical devices that cure, detect, or prevent diseases.

Funding Allocation by Institute and Center

The categorical research institutes and centers (hereinafter referred to as "institutes"), which have been established one by one over the years, have a variety of foci. Some are organized by disease or organ (e.g., cancer; alcoholism; deafness; heart, lung, and blood; eye; and dental). Some are based on stages of human development (e.g., aging and child health and human development). Some are organized by field of science and medicine (e.g., general medical sciences, environmental health, nursing, and human genome research). Other entities include the National Library of Medicine, John E. Fogarty International Center, and National Center for Research Resources. All of these institutes and centers report to the Office of the Director (see Figure 1-1).

There is a natural focus on the allocation of funding among the institutes and centers because each receives its own appropriation from Congress (the Office of the Director, Office of AIDS Research, and buildings and facilities accounts also receive separate appropriations; see Table C-1 in Appendix C).[1] The institutes and centers are the main organizational units of NIH, with only the Office of the Director of NIH being above them, providing overall leadership and direction and cross-institute coordination.[2]

---

[1]The Division of Research Grants (recently renamed the Center for Scientific Review), the Division of Computer Research and Technology (recently renamed the Center for Information Technology), and the Warren Grant Magnuson Clinical Center are funded through the NIH Management Fund, which is financed by "taps" on the institute and center appropriations.

[2]Even the Office of AIDS Research, although located in the Office of the Director of NIH, operates in many respects as an "institute without walls" with a director, national advisory council with scientific and public members (Office of AIDS Research Advisory Committee), an executive committee of senior program officials, and an executive office for staff support (Office of AIDS Research) (Institute of Medicine, 1991:42).

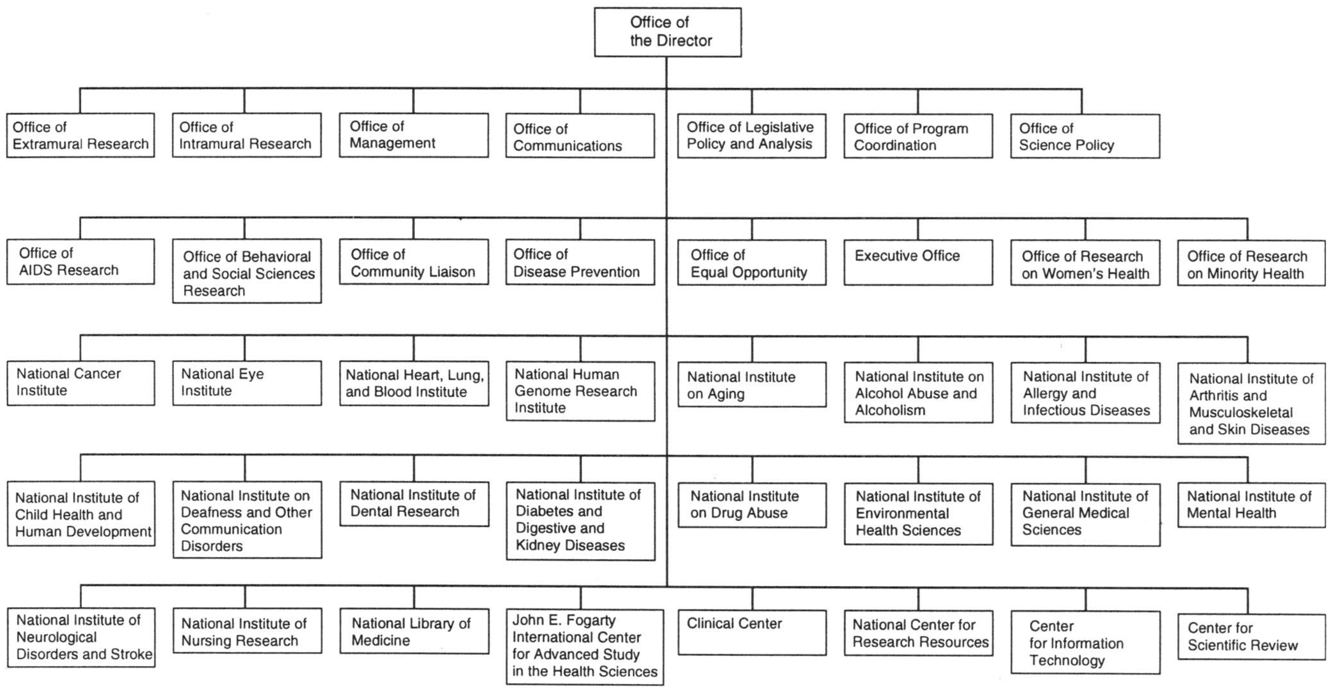

FIGURE 1-1 Organization of NIH. SOURCE: National Institutes of Health (1997d:13).

Each institute supports research, training, and information programs in its area. After research proposals from the nation's biomedical and behavioral scientists and engineers are peer reviewed for scientific merit, they are assigned to an institute for funding and administration. Most institutes and centers also have intramural programs.

Each institute is headed by a director who has strong research and leadership skills in the areas addressed by his or her institute. Each has a national advisory council with members representing the scientific community and the public to advise the institute director on policies and programs and to review and approve research grant applications. Institute directors are also advised on the intramural program by a Board of Scientific Counselors, consisting of nongovernment scientists with the appropriate expertise. The institutes are organized internally by research area, and the program heads also advise the directors on research priorities; in turn, they typically have standing and ad hoc advisory committees of nongovernment experts and, sometimes, public representatives (the standing advisory committees are listed by institute in Appendix A).

Funding Allocation by Mechanism

In its budget documents and presentations to Congress, after a table showing funding by institute, NIH usually presents a table or figure indicating funding by mechanism (see Table C-2 in Appendix C).[3] It indicates what share of NIH's budget goes to different mechanisms of support—for example, research project grants (RPGs), research and development (R&D) contracts, intramural research, and so forth. In FY 1998, for example, NIH expects to spend 56.7 percent ($7.7 billion) of its total budget on nearly 29,000 RPGs. RPGs are scientific studies or experiments proposed by researchers based in more than 1,700 universities, medical schools, and other research institutions in the United States and abroad.[4] About 8.8 percent of NIH's budget will go to support interdisciplinary research centers focused on a particular disease or other aspect of health, and 4.7 percent will go to support other types of research grants. R&D contracts will account for about 6.4 percent of NIH's budget, and intramural research at NIH itself will account for 10.4 percent of NIH's budget. Training of researchers will account for 3.1 percent of the NIH budget. The remainder will support program management and administration in the institutes, including the scientists and engineers who review research proposals and administer the extramural

[3]See, for example, the overview section of NIH's budget request to Congress (U.S. Department of Health and Human Services, 1998:62) or NIH's press release for its FY 1999 budget request (National Institutes of Health, 1998c).

[4]Almost two-thirds of RPGs are R01s, which support a single project proposed by a single principal scientist, NIH's most traditional form of support.

grant programs (3.6 percent), the Office of the Director of NIH (1.8 percent), the National Library of Medicine (1.2 percent), cancer control activities funded by NCI (1.9 percent), and construction of research facilities (1.7 percent).

NIH leaders monitor the allocation of funding among mechanisms because the levels of funding for different mechanisms of support help NIH to discern patterns in the nature of scientific work as well as detect changes in the balance between investigator-initiated and NIH-initiated work. As NIH's press release for its FY 1999 budget request put it, "NIH's highest priority is the funding of basic biomedical research through research project grants. The emphasis on peer-reviewed and competitively awarded RPGs allows NIH to sustain the scientific momentum of investigator-initiated research while providing new research opportunities" (National Institutes of Health, 1998a:7). NIH leaders focus particular attention on the number of new grants that can be awarded each year, because new grants constitute the part of NIH's budget that can be used most flexibly to address shifts in priorities, such as promising opportunities for new scientific advances, emerging health problems, or public health emergencies. Grant awards average 4 years. This multiyear funding is essential to the planning and conduct of successful investigations. It means that most of the annual RPG budget goes to continuing existing grants, which NIH calls its commitment base. In FY 1998, for example, more than 75 percent of the funding for RPGs is already committed and not quite 25 percent ($1.9 billion) is available for new projects.[5]

Other mechanisms, such as grants for research centers, clinical trials, and R&D contracts, tend to be more directed in nature and more tied to an institute's mission. They are usually solicited by NIH through requests for applications (RFAs) rather than initiated by extramural scientists, are reviewed by peer-review committees in the institutes rather than in the Center for Scientific Review, and are often funded as cooperative agreements in which NIH officials have more of a say in project direction than they do with RPGs. They also tend to be used more in problem-oriented research efforts, such as disease-specific programs, especially in their beginning stages (for example, in the early years of the War on Cancer and of research on AIDS and Alzheimer's disease). Because of their directedness, such mechanisms tend to be specified by Congress in legislation or report language when Congress concludes that NIH should move more quickly to attack a particular disease or other problem. If NIH's budget is increasing slowly, such mandates or set-asides for research centers, RFAs, or other specific mechanisms could impinge on the share of funding for investigator-initiated research projects.

---

[5]Some agencies that may fund multiyear grants (e.g., NSF) fully fund each grant up front rather than fund each grant incrementally year by year. Thus, 100 percent of each year's grant budget is potentially available for new priorities rather than the continuation of existing lines of research.

Funding Allocation by Type of Research

NIH also classifies its funding according to whether it is basic research, applied research, or development work, using definitions supplied by the federal Office of Management and Budget (OMB) for government-wide reporting purposes. Basic research is defined as "systematic study directed toward greater knowledge or understanding of the fundamental aspects of phenomena and of observable facts without specific applications towards processes or products in mind" (Office of Management and Budget, 1997). Applied research is "systematic study to gain knowledge or understanding necessary for determining the means by which a recognized and specific need may be met." Development is the "systematic application of knowledge toward the production of useful material, devices, and systems or methods, including design, development, and improvement of prototypes and new processes to meet specific requirements."

In FY 1998, excluding training, administration, and facilities, NIH expects about 57 percent of its budget to go to the support of basic research, 31 percent to applied research, and 12 percent to development (see Table C-3 in Appendix C).[6] Taken literally, these percentages mean that the majority of NIH funding is not immediately disease specific, because the research is so fundamental that the investigators do not know for certain which diseases their results might affect. No matter how esoteric their research may be, however, most if not all scientists are motivated by the fact that extending the frontiers of knowledge about basic biological and behavioral processes has greatly increased the current capacity to diagnose, treat, and prevent illnesses and enhance health and that it is virtually certain to do so in the future (although how or when cannot be predicted).

One should not take these percentages to be very precise, because in practice it is often difficult to classify research as basic or applied. For one thing, it involves determining whether the researcher has an application in mind. Even as rough estimates, however, the data indicate that, like other mission agencies of the federal government, NIH supports a substantial amount of basic research on the grounds that a growing science base will undoubtedly lead to better applications in the future.[7] History has proven this to be so. As noted in the previous section, however, NIH generally prefers to monitor the balance between research projects proposed by scientists and those proposed by NIH, as indicated by the mechanism of support. The rationale is that, on average, scientists working in laboratories across the country will have better ideas than NIH officials about where progress might be made, whether in basic or applied research.

---

[6]Calculated from information provided by NIH's Office of Financial Management.

[7]The percentages of R&D funding expected to go to basic research at other agencies in FY 1997 were 92 percent at NSF, 35 percent at the U.S. Department of Energy, 20 percent at the National Aeronautics and Space Administration, and 3 percent at the U.S. Department of Defense (National Science Foundation, 1997b:Table C-7).

Funding Allocation by Disease

NIH also keeps track of the annual amount of funding related to specific diseases and other particular purposes (see Table C-4 in Appendix C). These data have been kept for many years to enable NIH to respond to requests from Congress or others about how much it spends on "programs of interest." Most of the items are disease related, such as research on cancer, heart disease, stroke, AIDS, Alzheimer's disease, Parkinson's disease, diabetes, hepatitis C, and tuberculosis. Some focus on other categories of research, such as gene therapy, health and behavioral research, immunology, nutrition, prevention, rehabilitation, and vaccine development. Some concern research related to particular groups, such as research related to aging, pediatrics, the health of the rural populations, and women's health.

NIH tracks about 250 programs of interest and reports annually on about 50 of these. Some of the items included in the 50 change from year to year, depending on information requests. For example, in the FY 1999 appropriations hearings, NIH was asked about funding for research on a half-dozen programs (e.g., autism, food-borne illness, obesity, uterine and ovarian cancer, behavioral research, and international activities), and they will likely be included in the list next year.

The data are reported by each institute to NIH's Office of Financial Management, which means that it is possible to track funding by institute (see Tables C-5 and C-6 in Appendix C for funding for research on cancer and diabetes by institute, respectively). In some cases, institute-by-institute tables are reported regularly by the lead organization for a particular disease (e.g., the Office of AIDS Research and AIDS research or the National Institute on Aging and Alzheimer's disease).

In each institute, scientist-administrators review each grant and contract award and decide whether it is related to one or more of the programs of interest. In the case of a disease, they include more than just those awards that mention a disease in the title or in a list of key terms for inclusion in the computerized database system containing information on research projects and programs supported by NIH and other DHHS agencies. They also include basic research that is related because it is studying a phenomenon implicated in the disease. For example, research aimed at trying to gain a better understanding of the basic processes of neuronal death might be considered related to Alzheimer's disease. It would also probably be considered related to Parkinson's disease and some other neurodegenerative diseases marked by the progressive loss of neurons. At the same time, much basic research is too fundamental to be considered related to any specific disease. This means that some research is counted twice while other research is not counted at all in the data on funding by disease, even though the latter kind of research is helping to build the science base that will lead to the disease-specific advances of the future (see Box 1-3).

BOX 1-3 Basic Research Crosses Disease Boundaries

When establishing research priorities it is important to keep in mind that therapeutic advances frequently emerge from basic research that crosses disease boundaries. For example, much of the progress in AIDS treatment—including the blood test for AIDS and the protease inhibitors used to treat the disease—can be traced to the fundamental work of NIH-supported scientists who were researching cancer. In the 1960s and 1970s these scientists discovered certain viruses called retroviruses that cause cancer in chickens and mice. They learned an enormous amount about the biology of these viruses. Once it was discovered that the AIDS virus resembles a retrovirus, two decades of knowledge in the effort to study cancer could be applied to the understanding of AIDS. Building upon this base of knowledge derived from NIH-supported basic research in cancer, three companies simultaneously developed protease inhibitors for the treatment of AIDS.

Another crossover occurred between heart disease and cancer research. University scientists, supported by the National Heart, Lung, and Blood Institute, learned the fundamental mechanism for the regulation of cholesterol levels in blood. This allowed companies to develop drugs called statins that lower cholesterol levels and prevent heart attacks. Basic biologists, working on cancer, used the statins to discover a new property of cancer-causing proteins called Ras proteins. Pharmaceutical companies seized upon this information, and in 1998 they began clinical trials with new drugs that inactivate Ras proteins and thus may be useful in the treatment of cancer. All of this progress in cancer treatment is directly traceable to the discovery of statins through NIH's program of basic research in heart disease.

In the table of spending by disease in its budget submission to Congress and on its web page, NIH does not provide population-based information such as the number of people who are afflicted or who die annually or cost-of-illness estimates. The institutes with lead responsibility for particular diseases sometimes collect and publish information on burden of disease and economic costs, but they use different databases and methodologies, which limit the comparability of their results.

Despite limitations, these data are used by health groups and advocates to help assess how much effort NIH is putting into research on particular diseases, that is, as a measure of NIH priority setting. Disease-specific interest groups usually report on the rate of increase in funding for research on the disease in which they are interested and compare it with those for research on other diseases, and they may compare spending per afflicted person to argue that NIH is neglecting the disease in which they are interested. Some members of Congress have also used the data to judge whether the allocation of NIH funding matches the burdens and costs of diseases in the population. These issues are discussed in Chapter 2, where there is further analysis of the reporting system and recommendations for improving it.

RECENT TRENDS AND ISSUES

NIH is the leading federal agency supporting research related to improving the nation's health. By various key measures it has been very successful in fulfilling its mission. The scientists and clinicians whom it has helped train and whose research careers it has supported have consistently been in the forefront of research discoveries that have advanced fundamental knowledge of human biology and of better ways to treat or prevent disease and promote good health. Over the past 50 years NIH as an institution has played a substantial role in contributing to the explosion of knowledge that has amounted to a revolution in biology. One indicator of NIH's contributions to science is the number of Nobel Prize-winning scientists and physicians whom it has supported. Over the years NIH has funded 93 Nobel Prize winners for work ranging from deciphering the genetic code to determining the cause of diseases to developing better techniques to diagnose, treat, or prevent diseases. There are many examples of how NIH-supported work has contributed to better medical care and health. They include the decline in the rate of mortality from heart disease, the leading cause of death in the United States, by nearly 50 percent over the past 20 years. Death rates from stroke decreased by 50 percent during the same period. Dental sealants have sharply reduced the number of cavities in children.

Despite tremendous progress, however, there is still a long way to go in conquering disease. At the same time, the benefits of past research have not reached everyone, as indicated by significant differentials in disease rates and outcomes among members of different socioeconomic and ethnic groups. Demographic trends will have an impact; for example, the aging of the population will substantially increase the individual and social burdens of certain diseases and conditions. Also, about half the nation's health care costs result from unhealthy behaviors and environments, which pose major research challenges (McGinnis and Foege, 1993).

NIH's success has earned it steady budget increases despite a tight overall federal budget in recent years. The NIH budget is $13.6 billion in FY 1998, and the administration has proposed an increase of 8.4 percent to $14.7 billion in FY 1999. Some members of Congress have talked about a larger increase. Despite the favorable budget trend (NIH's budget has increased by 80 percent since 1990, compared with an increase of 48 percent in the rest of the nondefense discretionary budget), concern about research priority setting at NIH has grown in recent years. For example, since 1995 there have been at least eight instances in which members of Congress or congressional committees have asked about priority setting in some aspect of NIH's research program, not including the one leading to this report.[8]

Concerns about priority setting in the allocation of NIH research funding come from several sources. First, some members of Congress believe that there should be more of a correlation between the allocation of funding by disease and the distribution of disease burdens and costs in the population. They point to widely different amounts of research funding per afflicted person from one disease to another and ask why NIH is spending much more per death from HIV/AIDS infections compared with spending per death from cancer, from heart disease, and from stroke. They also note that the largest amounts of NIH funding do not always go toward research on diseases that cost the federal government the most through the Medicare program (see, for example, the charts and discussion in U.S. Congress [1997a:36–42] and Agnew [1996]).

Second, more and more disease-specific interest groups have begun campaigning for increases in NIH funding for research related to the particular diseases in which they are interested. They are urging Congress to set aside specific amounts by disease or to boost the funding for the institute that supports most of the research on their disease of interest relative to that for other institutes. They point to the amount of funding related to their disease of interest, compare it with the larger amounts being devoted to other diseases, and question the priority-setting process that led to that result. Traditionally, disease-specific interest groups have avoided open competition with each other for NIH funding. Rather, they supported increases generally for NIH, expecting to benefit from the overall increase, perhaps lobbying quietly to win a larger than average increase for their program or institute. The success of the direct approach for some groups, however, has put pressure on all groups to make more specific demands and to compete openly with other groups for more resources.

Third, the leadership of the health committees in Congress has become increasingly uncomfortable with intervening in research priority setting at NIH, for example, by mandating specific funding set-asides, new programs or institutions focused on a specific disease, or the use of particular research mechanisms or by trying to push research advances in specific areas in other ways. In part they may be reacting to feedback about the unintended effects of disease-specific earmarking in the late 1980s and early 1990s that added up to more than the overall increases and thus cut into the funding for other programs (Congress has always included earmarks in report language or less formally, but until recently, they rarely added up to a substantial share of the total budget increase that NIH received in any given year and so did not affect other research areas directly). They are also facing a large and growing set of groups pushing for earmarks, making it even harder to satisfy such demands within the overall

[8]From a list provided by the NIH Office of Legislative Policy and Analysis.

increases. NIH leaders and the scientific community also began to object strongly to overly detailed prescriptions about priority setting and funding allocations from Congress. The director of NIH and the institute directors have testified on a number of occasions that congressional directives "distort" the priority-setting process because they do not allow NIH to adjust for the different probabilities of scientific progress against each health problem and because they do not properly weigh the need for basic research for progress in the long run (the director and several institute directors made this point to the IOM committee at the committee's first meeting on March 6, 1998) (see also Varmus [1997] and the testimony of Harold Varmus, director of NIH [U.S. House of Representatives, 1997a; U.S. Senate, 1997a]).

In the markup of the Senate reauthorization bill, the NIH Revitalization Act of 1996, members of the authorization committee began to debate whether Congress should be directive by authorizing more set-asides for specific diseases or should let NIH determine the direction for research funding. They were considering a number of amendments that authorized specific funding amounts and mandated certain mechanisms for particular diseases (U.S. Senate, 1996:10; also see the section on the 1996 Senate Reauthorization Bill in Chapter 5).

The 1996 reauthorization effort had many members of the Senate authorization subcommittee saying that they "should not micromanage biomedical research by establishing legislative mandates for specific areas" (U.S. Senate, 1997a:10). One result was that the subcommittee held an important hearing in May 1997 on research priority setting at NIH (U.S. Senate, 1997a).[9] The subcommittee heard testimony from the director of NIH and representatives of the scientific community in universities and industry who strongly encouraged Congress to resist pressures to become involved in how much NIH should spend on research targeted to specific diseases (see, for example, testimony by John W. Suttie, president of the Federation of American Societies for Experimental Biology [U.S. Senate, 1997a:59–60]). Representatives of voluntary organizations promoting health research testified that one reason that disease-specific interest groups appeal directly to Congress for earmarks or set-asides is the perceived lack of opportunities to be consulted in the planning and priority-setting process at NIH (see testimony by Myrl Weinberg, president, National Health Council [U.S. Senate, 1997a:63–64]).

Questions about the desirability of congressional micromanagement were also being raised on the House side. In an oversight hearing held by the House authorization subcommittee in September 1997, Congressman Greg Ganske discussed the issue (U.S. House of Representatives, 1997b:4):

> I do have significant concerns about whether Congress has played politics with the NIH budget and micromanaged difficult scientific questions. . . . While

---

[9]Two more Senate hearings were held on specific issues (see U.S. Senate, 1997b,c).

> promoting an increase in funding for one disease or another, I am concerned that these lobbying efforts are turning the floor of Congress into a scientific peer review panel. We are being asked whether to spend additional millions on breast cancer or diabetes or Parkinson's, and the list goes on and on. . . . I have concerns about whether members of Congress have the scientific expertise to determine where the most promising areas of research are.

By September 1997, the campaign by groups advocating for increased research on Parkinson's disease succeeded when the Senate voted to include the Udall Bill authorizing a $100 million program consisting of research centers, training grants, a patient information center, and other mechanisms in the FY 1998 appropriations bill. Advocates had argued that NIH had neglected Parkinson's disease research in terms of the burden and cost of the disease and scientific opportunities and that Congress should take active steps to correct the disparity (see, for example, funding comparison charts and written testimony by Joan I. Samuelson, president, Parkinson's Action Network [U.S. Senate, 1997a:76–80]). In speeches on the Senate floor when the amendment for the Udall Bill was being debated, leaders of the authorization committee expressed concern over the process by which Congress mandated programs piecemeal in response to organized lobbying efforts. They proposed that IOM conduct an independent study of NIH's priority-setting process that would recommend any changes needed so that Congress could rely on NIH to make the allocation decisions (see speeches by Senators Dan Coats and Bill Frist [U.S. Congress, 1997b:S8714–S8716]). That proposal led to the present study and asked IOM to pay particular attention to two features: NIH's mechanisms for public input and the role of Congress in directing the allocation of funding among areas of research.

IOM COMMITTEE PROCESS

The IOM committee proceeded by assessing NIH's priority-setting process in light of the agency's mission and objectives and the changing policy environment. The committee addressed the following questions in the charge: Are the criteria adequate? Is the process for implementing them working? Given the objective of responding to health needs as well as scientific opportunity, in conjunction with the expansion of organized disease-specific interest groups, are the mechanisms for public input adequate or can they be changed to increase the complementarity between NIH's goals of responding to health needs and scientific opportunity? Can Congress, the holder of the public purse strings, be assured that NIH has a good process for priority setting in which the full range of considerations is taken into account in planning programs and allocating funding?

In an effort to be as comprehensive as possible in the short time allowed, the committee pursued several mechanisms for collecting data and receiving input. At the committee's request, NIH provided a large amount of data regarding its research programs and budgetary and priority-setting processes. These data included organizational information, funding histories, and descriptions of the priority-setting processes in each institute at NIH. The committee also held organized panel discussions with the NIH director and deputy director, the directors of institutes and offices at NIH, and congressional staff. In addition, the committee solicited and received public comment through presentations and panel discussions at a public meeting, via a questionnaire mailed to more than 1,000 NIH constituency groups, and through the committee's web site.

The committee felt that it was important to receive as much input as possible from public groups involved with or seeking involvement in NIH's research priority-setting process. To do so, the committee convened a public meeting on April 3, 1998, to gather information and hear from groups or individuals, especially those identified by the NIH institutes as being part of their constituencies. The committee made every effort to include as many groups as possible, given the short time available.

Twenty-nine patient-advocacy groups and professional societies appeared before the committee (see Appendix B) in panels and an open comment session. Although each participant had a unique perspective, several themes became evident:

- Many presenters felt that research funding should reflect, among other factors, the burden of disease in society. The difficulty of this approach becomes apparent, however, when considering rare diseases. Although NIH indicates that it takes disease burden into account, several panelists felt that the criteria that NIH uses to set research priorities are unclear or ambiguous.
- Many advocacy groups are familiar with NIH and its organizational structure, but for issues that cross institute lines or for which there is no precedent, groups can find themselves at a loss about where to turn.
- There is a need for greater patient or public representation on NIH advisory bodies.
- There is a need for better communication between NIH and constituency groups.

The committee received written comments from 56 individuals and organizations (including those from panelists at the committee's public meeting [see Appendix B]). These comments came from a spectrum of individuals involved with NIH—from researchers and advisers to patient-advocates and patients themselves—on issues ranging from education and training to disease-specific allocations of funding for research. The comments addressed many different topics or elements of the priority-setting process. Many called for more research funding allocations for specific diseases; others requested added emphases on certain types of research, such as environmental, interdisciplinary, clinical, or basic research. Still others commented that Congress should play a different role in priority setting, including some who believed that it should have greater involvement and some who believed that it should have less involvement. Many commentators noted the importance of increased inclusiveness in the identification of health research needs and highlighted the importance of open communication.

ORGANIZATION OF THE REPORT

The remainder of this report is organized into sections that address issues related to criteria for priority setting (Chapter 2), priority-setting processes (Chapter 3), mechanisms for public input (Chapter 4), and the role of the U.S. Congress (Chapter 5). Several appendixes (A to D) are included, as follows: Appendix A, Federal Advisory Committees of NIH; Appendix B, Acknowledgments; Appendix C, NIH funding tables; and Appendix D, committee and staff biographies.

2

Criteria for Priority Setting

The first charge to the committee was "to assess the factors or criteria used by NIH to determine funding allocations for disease research." The committee defined the charge broadly to include the adequacy of the criteria used to set priorities and allocate resources among all areas of research, some but not all of which are disease specific, in order to fulfill the mission of NIH to improve health through research.

WHY CRITERIA ARE IMPORTANT

NIH's budget for the current FY (1998) of $13.6 billion makes it the largest civilian research agency in the federal government (accounting for 37 percent of the federal nondefense R&D budget). Nevertheless, there is never as much funding as is needed to address all important health problems and pursue all research opportunities or as much funding as NIH's supporters would like it to have. Choices must be made and priorities must be set.

Priorities are not only driven by a scarcity of resources. They are also affected by health emergencies and epidemics, demographic trends affecting health, such as the aging of the population or changing patterns of tobacco and alcohol use, and new opportunities in science stemming from research advances or better research instruments.

The criteria that guide these choices are essential for public understanding of NIH's activities and for ensuring adequate levels of public support for its mission and budget. These criteria are a key element in the agency's accountability to the public.

How NIH allocates funding among areas of research has become a major issue over the past several years. As noted in Chapter 1, Congress has inquired about priorities among specific diseases or programs on a number of occasions since 1995. Some legislators believe that the distribution of NIH funding does not adequately reflect the number of citizens affected by various diseases or the costs of various diseases to society. Advocates for individuals with various diseases tell Congress that NIH is neglecting research on their focal disease relative to the levels of research on other diseases. Congress has also become concerned about how NIH allocates funding to areas that are not disease specific, for example, clinical research (versus basic research) and public health education.

NIH'S CRITERIA FOR PRIORITY SETTING

In response to concerns about how it allocates funding among categories of research, NIH recently published "Setting Research Priorities at the National Institutes of Health," a 15-page booklet describing the criteria and processes that it currently uses (National Institutes of Health, 1997b) (referred to hereafter as Setting Research Priorities). In its FY 1999 budget request, NIH told Congress that the booklet "delineated" NIH's priority-setting principles and mechanisms and that NIH would "continue to consider the full array of relevant criteria in setting priorities for research funding, including the societal and economic costs associated with particular diseases and disorders" (U.S. Department of Health and Human Services, 1998:OD-33).

Setting Research Priorities lists five major general criteria that NIH calls "both influential and continuous" in priority setting (National Institutes of Health, 1997b:4). These criteria are

- public health needs,
- scientific quality of the research,
- potential for scientific progress (the existence of promising pathways and qualified investigators),
- portfolio diversification along the broad and expanding frontiers of research, and
- adequate support of infrastructure (human capital, equipment and instrumentation, and facilities).

According to NIH, these criteria are used to set priorities in a broad and complicated program with multiple goals and numerous levels. They are used in a process that allocates funding among NIH institutes and centers and, within each institute or center, among a hierarchy of programs. These allocation choices affect how much goes to basic versus clinical versus epidemiologic research, to need-driven versus science-driven research, to intramural versus extramural programs, to solicited versus investigator-initiated research projects, and to specific mechanisms, such as grants to investigator-proposed projects, grants solicited by NIH through specific RFAs, contracts, and centers, and so forth. They also affect the allocation of research funding among disease-specific activities on the one hand and more general or crosscutting activities on the other (e.g., research on basic processes that underlie many or all diseases and the research infrastructure).

Decision making—that is, priority setting—is highly decentralized at NIH, as is appropriate for a research organization with diverse forms of specialized expertise. However, the cumulative impact of such decisions needs to be monitored and perhaps adjusted at each level, especially at the level of the institute directors and the level of the director of NIH. That will ensure that priorities that involve higher-level coordination are met, that there are no significant gaps or unnecessary overlaps in research, and that emerging problems and opportunities affecting NIH and its mission are recognized. These process issues are addressed in Chapter 3. This chapter addresses the adequacy and completeness of the criteria per se (listed in National Institutes of Health [1997b:4]).

Criterion 1. Public Health Needs

> *The NIH has an obligation to respond to public health needs, as judged by the incidence, severity, and cost of specific disorders. Calculating these needs is difficult, and there is not always clear distinction between expense and results* (National Institutes of Health, 1997b:4).

Public health needs is clearly an important priority-setting criterion for an agency with the mission of uncovering new knowledge that will lead to better health for everyone. However, the description of the response to public health needs quoted above from Setting Research Priorities as being related to addressing specific disorders is too narrow. It reduces the concept of health to the absence of disease instead of taking a broader view of health as leading a full and high-quality life even in the presence of pathologies, chronic symptoms, and functional limitations (Institute of Medicine, 1997). NIH's actual research portfolio reflects this broader conception of health. Research on the needs of persons with disabling conditions, for example, focuses on treatment but also on how factors in the environment can be modified to enable them to function more fully despite their pathology.

In 1995, at the request of Congress, NIH published a report with a table listing the burdens and costs of 66 diseases and conditions, including the 15 leading causes of death, and the amount of research funding that NIH was devoting to each. The data in that report and a later edition with more recent data

(National Institutes of Health, 1997a) have been used by critics of NIH priority setting to argue that there is little correlation between the distribution of disease burdens or costs and NIH funding allocations, for example, by finding much higher research spending per death from relatively rare diseases compared with the leading causes of death (see Table C-7 in Appendix C for an excerpt from the table in the report). NIH for its part notes that the data were derived in different ways and at different times, which limits comparability, that cost-of-illness studies have serious methodological limitations, and that even if the data were improved, many other important factors would have to be taken into account in allocating research dollars, such as the importance of research advances and opportunities and the availability of research tools and trained personnel (National Institutes of Health, 1997a:4–5).

Setting Research Priorities discusses alternative indicators of public health needs in greater detail in a later section on assessing health needs (National Institutes of Health, 1997b:8–9). It notes that U.S. health needs indicators that could be considered in allocating research funds include

- number of people who have a particular disease;
- number of deaths caused by a disease;
- degree of disability produced by a disease;
- degree to which a disease cuts short a normal, productive, comfortable life;
- economic and social costs of a disease; and
- need to act rapidly to control the spread of a disease.

Setting Research Priorities notes that all these criteria are relevant and, conversely, that the use of any one of these criteria exclusively would lead to the unwarranted neglect of some diseases (National Institutes of Health, 1997b). For example, "funding according to the number of deaths would neglect chronic diseases that produce long-term disability and high costs to society (disease such as mental illness and arthritis would be neglected)," but "funding according to the economic cost of illness would under-fund diseases that result in short illness and rapid death (this choice would result in a great deal of funding for Alzheimer's disease and muscular dystrophy and little, or none, for sudden infant death syndrome or certain types of cancer)" (p. 9). Moreover, the booklet says, "any of these criteria used exclusively would . . . underfund research on rare diseases, research that has taught us much about the diseases themselves and a great deal about normal human biology, other diseases, and new approaches to treatment" (p. 9).

NIH's discussion of these indicators reflects the recognition that the selection of measures is an expression of values (National Research Council, 1996), insofar as each will increase the priority placed on some health problems and decrease that placed on others. The booklet does not describe, however, how NIH in practice combines these (or other) health indicators in setting its research priorities or how these indicators are integrated with the other criteria, such as the degree of scientific opportunity, when allocating resources among programs or creating new programs.

Nor does NIH have a systematic process for collecting and analyzing data on the full range of health indicators (e.g., demographic trends and societal changes), whether on its own or through arrangements with agencies that do, such as the Health Care Financing Administration and the National Center for Health Statistics, Centers for Disease Control and Prevention. As a result, it is not in a position to evaluate its success in meeting this criterion. For example, changes in the age structure of the nation's population and the growth in the numbers of people who are members of minority groups and of persons with disabling conditions have important implications for the incidence and prevalence of certain health problems. NIH's current informal arrangements for considering health needs indicators leave it open to charges that it only gives lip service to consideration of the broad spectrum of health needs in setting priorities and allocating resources.

As noted in Chapter 1, NIH's Office of Financial Management has long tracked how much it spends on particular diseases and other activities to be able to respond to inquiries from Congress and other interested groups and individuals (see Table C-4 in Appendix C). Disease-specific interest groups use these statistics to help assess the priority that NIH gives to particular diseases or health problems relative to the priorities that it gives to other diseases or problems. In so doing, these groups are in effect trying to figure out NIH's implicit policy for implementing Criterion 1. However, NIH's position is that little reliance should be placed on these numbers because of variations in definitions and accounting procedures from institute to institute and over time. Indeed, although the Office of Financial Management has provided standard definitions for approximately 30 of the approximately 250 categories for which it compiles data reported by the institutes, it does not have the resources to ensure consistency and quality (the Office of Financial Management staff levels have been cut by two-thirds in recent years). In any case, such revealed preferences analyses (as economists would describe attempts to infer priorities from observed behavior) are a poor substitute for the direct expression of NIH's priorities and documentation and for the evaluation of their implementation. Nor can they capture the contribution of basic biological or behavioral research that could contribute to reducing multiple health problems.

In assessing public health needs as a factor in the process of allocating funds, NIH also must consider the disease-specific research being supported by others, including industry, voluntary health associations, and foundations. The combined research budgets of pharmaceutical companies and biotechnology firms are greater than that of NIH and are largely concentrated on applied research and development of new drugs and other disease-specific products. NIH should not fund research that would be supported by industry.

Criterion 2. Quality of Research Supported

> *The NIH applies stringent review for scientific quality on all research proposals in order to return the maximum possible on the public's investment in medical research* (National Institutes of Health, 1997b:4).

The text of this criterion reflects NIH's long-standing reliance on peer review of specific research proposals by relevant scientific experts to ensure that it supports the best projects in terms of scientific impact or significance, technical merit and feasibility, researcher qualifications, and facility adequacy. Although scientific peer review of each proposal is an important part of NIH's success, it relies on specialized criteria and processes that are not the main focus of this report. This report looks at the process that determines how funding is allocated *among* the various research programs, not how specific proposals are chosen for funding *within* each research program.

The committee is aware that NIH has undertaken a major revamping of the peer-review process. The Division of Research Grants created in 1948 was elevated to the Center for Scientific Review in 1997 and was placed under new leadership. The review criteria and process used by the Center for Scientific Review have been assessed by several groups, most recently, the Peer Review Oversight Group, a panel appointed by the director of NIH. The Peer Review Oversight Group recommended revised criteria, which have been adopted (see Box 2-1).

NIH is also addressing another problem in the peer-review system: the poor success of clinical research proposals competing for approval with basic research proposals within research areas addressed by review groups (called study sections). The problem, which is linked to the decline in the number of clinical investigators in recent years, was identified in several studies, including one by an IOM committee (Institute of Medicine, 1994). The NIH Director's Panel on Clinical Research recommended changes in its December 1997 report (NIH Director's Panel on Clinical Research, 1997), such as increasing the percentage of clinical research proposals to 30 to 50 percent in those sections reviewing them and increasing the number of experienced clinicians on those study sections, increasing support for training and research support programs for clinical investigators, and expanding the General Clinical Research Center program of the National Center for Research Resources (National Institutes of Health, 1997c).

The director of the Center for Scientific Review recently appointed a blue ribbon external panel to address the aspect of peer review that most affects overall priority setting among study sections: the NIH practice of "percentiling," that is, funding the same percentage of proposals in each study section, which means that each section has a certain claim on funding. As a result, the allocation of funding among research topics is affected in part by the structure of the study sections. If the structure does not keep up with changes in science—that is, if study sections are not created and phased out as the frontiers of science advance and scientific fields become obsolete and new ones emerge—then the allocation of the majority of NIH's funding that goes through the Center for Scientific Review is adversely affected. The new blue ribbon panel was directed explicitly to address this problem and recommend ways to update and to keep updated the study section structure.

BOX 2-1 NIH Peer-Review Criteria for Individual Investigator-Initiated Research Project Proposals

Significance: Does this study address an important problem? If the aims of the application are achieved, how will scientific knowledge be advanced? What will be the effect of these studies on the concepts or methods that drive this field?

Approach: Are the conceptual framework, design, methods, and analyses adequately developed, well integrated, and appropriate to the aims of the project? Does the applicant acknowledge potential problem areas and consider alternative tactics?

Innovation: Does the project employ novel concepts, approaches, or methods? Are the aims original and innovative? Does the project challenge existing paradigms or develop new methodologies or technologies?

Investigator: Is the investigator appropriately trained and well suited to carry out this work? Is the proposed work appropriate to the experience levels of the principal investigator and other researchers (if any)?

Environment: Does the scientific environment in which the work will be done contribute to the probability of success? Do the proposed experiments take advantage of unique features of the scientific environment or employ useful collaborative arrangements? Is there evidence of institutional support?

In addition to the above criteria, in accordance with NIH policy, all applications will also be reviewed with respect to the following:

- The adequacy of plans to include as subjects members of both genders and of minority groups and their subgroups as appropriate for the scientific goals of the research. Plans for the recruitment and retention of subjects will also be evaluated.
- The reasonableness of the proposed budget and duration in relation to the proposed research.
- The adequacy of the proposed protection for humans, animals, or the environment, to the extent that they may be adversely affected by the project proposed in the application.

Criterion 3. Scientific Opportunity

> *As an administrator of science, the NIH has learned that many significant advances occur when new findings, often unforeseen, expand experimental possibilities and open new pathways for the imagination. Not all problems are equally approachable, no matter their importance to public health. Pursuit of a rare disease may often have unexpected benefits for more common problems. By the same token, increased spending on a disease is wasteful when there are neither promising pathways to follow nor an adequate number of qualified investigators to fund* (National Institutes of Health, 1997b:4).

Setting Research Priorities has an extended discussion of assessing scientific opportunities (National Institutes of Health, 1997b:10–11), which notes that it "is no less complex than evaluating health needs":

> It requires expertise in various scientific fields, breadth of vision across many disciplines, and judgment to determine the likely yield from making investments in particular areas of research. It is never known with certainty which scientific areas will produce the greatest returns soonest. At any given time, moreover, some fields are judged to be progressing more rapidly than others and more likely to repay the investment in them by yielding great discoveries that advance knowledge.

This discussion touches on two aspects of scientific discovery. First, at any given time, some areas of research are more promising than others because, for example, recent advances open new lines of inquiry or a new instrument makes it feasible to explore long-standing research questions for the first time. This situation is addressed by the scientific opportunity criterion. Second, other discoveries are serendipitous or turn out to have effects in areas that seemed remotely related at first. This is addressed by the next criterion, portfolio diversification.

NIH has well-established and elaborate procedures, described in Chapter 3, for assessing scientific merit in priority setting beginning with the expertise of its own staff and strongly supplemented by formal and ad hoc mechanisms for receiving advice from outside experts. The committee wants to ensure that, in NIH's decision making on programs and funding of research, NIH has adequate procedures to ensure scientific innovation and to foster support for high-risk research with high payoffs if it is successful, interdisciplinary research that crosses program and study group lines, and unconventional but promising research approaches. Some of the institutes have adopted procedures and programs for ensuring innovative research, and as noted above, innovation has been explicitly added to the list of peer-review criteria.

Criterion 4. Portfolio Diversification

> *The NIH's portfolio must be large and diverse. Because we cannot predict discoveries or anticipate the opportunities fresh discoveries will produce, the NIH must support research along a broad—in fact, expanding—frontier* (National Institutes of Health, 1997b:4).

Although it may invest differentially in areas of scientific promise, NIH also tries to invest in every health-related area of research to some degree. This prudent strategy is a hedge against the uncertainty of knowing where some if not most advances will actually occur, especially in the long run.

Each of the NIH institutes also funds a continuum of research approaches, from basic inquiries to clinical applications. "By supporting disease-related and basic research projects simultaneously, the NIH can achieve both near-term improvements in the diagnosis, treatment, and prevention of specific diseases as well as long-term discoveries in basic science that in time will produce great advances in our ability to understand, treat, and prevent disease or delay its onset" (National Institutes of Health, 1997b:9).

NIH could put all of its resources into applying current knowledge to health problems. Unfortunately, current knowledge is usually inadequate to lead to complete prevention of or cures for many diseases and conditions, although in many cases it may lead to better diagnosis and treatment or prevention options. Alternatively, NIH could invest all of its resources into long-term basic research to build the knowledge base for complete cures or prevention. This approach would leave those suffering now with no benefit from what knowledge is available, and it would not create the needed bridges from the laboratory to the real world, nor would it allow basic research to be informed systematically by clinical experience.

Although NIH should, and does, invest in the full range of research approaches (e.g., basic, translational, clinical, epidemiologic, and behavioral research), the balance among them should depend on the state of knowledge in each problem area. At its public hearing and in written submissions, the committee received testimony that certain fields of research (e.g., clinical, social, and behavioral research) are not given enough priority within NIH's overall research portfolio.

NIH is aware of this issue. The report and recommendations of the NIH Director's Panel on Clinical Research have already been discussed. The Office of Behavioral and Social Research in the Office of the Director of NIH was established in 1993 to foster greater attention to the social and behavioral aspects of health-related research. In establishing both the panel and the office, however, NIH acted only after receiving explicit directives from Congress.

Criterion 5. Adequate Infrastructure Support

> *The NIH must continue to support the human capital and material assets of science. To this end, the NIH's budget supports research training, acquisition of equipment and instruments, some limited construction projects, and grantee institutions' costs of enabling the research programs* (National Institutes of Health, 1997b:4).

Finally, NIH must invest in the long-term integrity of the health research enterprise, not just the costs of current research projects. As an earlier IOM committee concluded, "the most critical and longest-term investment in the research system is the development of career scientists who contribute to the long-term success of the enterprise through both their own research efforts and their training of future generations of scientists" (Institute of Medicine, 1990:5). That committee also concluded that capital investment in adequate facilities and equipment was another necessary long-term investment. These bases of a strong research system must be developed or increased investment in research projects will have less of an impact.

Furthermore, a major change in the ethnic makeup of the nation is taking place. It is essential that NIH invest in training members of growing minority groups, because it directly affects the health of those communities. These communities offer a perspective that would enrich the research enterprise and improve priority setting. Outreach to and involvement of members of minority communities in training programs will also help make those communities part of the biomedical research system.

CONCLUSIONS AND RECOMMENDATIONS

The testimony that the committee heard at its open meeting on April 3, 1998, or that it received in written form indicates that disease-specific interest groups are generally satisfied with NIH's priority-setting criteria, although they are not necessarily satisfied with how the criteria are applied in practice (an issue addressed in Chapter 3 on priority-setting processes).

In its discussions, the committee concluded that NIH's criteria for priority setting are reasonable and appropriate. Use of these criteria has been one of the most important factors contributing to the great success of NIH; the balanced application of these criteria has led to the accumulation of basic knowledge about human biology that is unparalleled in the history of science. This increased understanding has, in turn, led to better approaches to the diagnosis, prevention, and treatment of disease. However, the conceptualization of public health needs (Criterion 1) should be broadened beyond the medical model implied in the discussion of the criterion in Setting Research Priorities. Improving health through research goes beyond treating diseases to understanding how to promote healthy lifestyles and help those with diseases and disabilities improve their quality of life, and NIH in fact already supports such research. The committee also wants to ensure that the concept of human resources in the infrastructure criterion (Criterion 5) include outreach to underrepresented groups in biomedical and behavioral research careers.

> ***Recommendation 1.* The committee generally supports the criteria that NIH uses for priority setting and recommends that NIH continue to use these criteria in a balanced way to cover the full spectrum of research related to human health.**

By beginning to elucidate these criteria, NIH has provided a potentially valuable tool for all those concerned with its priority-setting operations. Members of any group may now look to see whether their goals appear in this statement of NIH's philosophy and what weight they are afforded. To the extent that the criteria are made clear and thus understandable to members of the public, citizens can examine NIH's procedures to see if they are consonant with these stated criteria, and they can assess NIH's actions to see how well this philosophy has been realized in practice. For NIH staff, these criteria will provide guidance as they establish and implement procedures as well as when they report on their activities and accomplishments. Over time the criteria could provide clear, predictable goals for their aspirations and standards for their accountability.

> ***Recommendation 2.* NIH should make clear its mechanisms for implementing its criteria for setting priorities and should evaluate their use and effectiveness.**

NIH's public health needs criterion requires systematic analysis of its portfolio in terms of public health statistics. There may be no simple relationship between health statistics (especially any single measure) and how NIH allocates funding. However, NIH should be able to show that it has considered data on health burdens and costs in a systematic fashion, in addition to considering scientific opportunity, cost differences among different kinds of research, non-NIH investments in health-related research (e.g., investments by industry, other government agencies, philanthropic institutions, and other countries), and other relevant factors. Some institutes conduct regular analyses of disease rates both to adjust future research agendas to changing trends and to assess the impacts of past research advances.* Such analyses might be done more systematically across NIH. NIH has also compiled statistics in response to specific congressional requests (National Institutes of Health, 1997a). What is called for here is a regular process that is supported by a clear philosophy and that is sensitive to

---

*For example, see the recent report on trends in cancer rates (Wingo et al., 1998).

scientific understanding of the meaning of such data and their interpretation (National Research Council, 1996).

> ***Recommendation 3.*** **In setting priorities, NIH should strengthen its analysis and use of health data, such as burdens and costs of diseases, and of data on the impact of research on the health of the public.**

Individuals and groups concerned about specific health problems or health research often use NIH-generated data on spending by specific disease or area of research to assess the overall research portfolio. Because NIH officials have said that NIH's own statistics on spending by disease are not very useful, it is incumbent on those officials to improve the quality and analysis of its data on the allocation of NIH funds by disease for planning and priority-setting purposes. NIH could approach the problem by being more systematic about deciding what to track and publish, using consistent definitions, deciding how much "related" as well as "direct" research should be included, keeping the statistics current, and ensuring quality control.

NIH should enhance its efforts at communicating and explaining the data to the public. For example, calculations of spending by disease should include not only all research directly related to the disease but also research projects on fundamental areas indirectly related to that disease. Users of the data should know that such calculations reflect the best estimates of total NIH spending in particular areas and that fundamental science is essential to discovering the etiology and progression of disease and other basic knowledge needed to develop improved means of diagnosis, improved prevention efforts, and improved treatments.

In making this recommendation, the committee is mindful of the limits on the use of such data in research priority setting. Health needs is an important factor, but there is rarely a straightforward one-to-one relationship between health needs and research funding allocations. This is shown in NIH's discussion of the limits to simple measures of health needs, as well as the need to consider other criteria. For example, the scientific opportunities for progress vary greatly across diseases in terms of the knowledge base, promising lines of inquiry, and the availability of sufficient numbers of researchers and facilities. Therefore, the amount of research support that can be linked directly to a specific disease is not by itself an adequate measure of how much or how well NIH is making progress against that disease. Nor does it reflect the potential relevance of basic research to specific diseases (e.g., research on dopamine receptors or transporters are relevant to Parkinson's disease and other diseases, even though the disease may not be mentioned in the title of the grants). As a result, NIH should improve its mechanisms for analyzing such connections to help ensure that the potential relevance of basic research to specific diseases is understood and capitalized upon.

NIH should also collect and analyze data on health research spending by others, such as other federal agencies, industry, nonprofit health organizations that fund research, foundations, or other countries. This should help identify gaps, overlaps, and opportunities for joint efforts and ensure that NIH invests wisely in areas and approaches that no one else is funding, provides the appropriate coordination, and supports the training of personnel and the other infrastructure needed in the national research enterprise.

> ***Recommendation 4.* NIH should improve the quality and analysis of its data on funding by disease and should include both direct and related expenditures.**

The full and adequate implementation of Recommendations 3 and 4—to improve data collection and analysis both within NIH and in collaboration with other agencies and the private sector—will require more resources and personnel, which should be considered necessary costs, much as the costs of the peer-review process are. The need for additional resources for priority setting is addressed to Congress in Recommendation 12, which addresses current congressional limitations on research management and support budgets.

3

Priority-Setting Processes

The second charge to the committee was to "assess the process by which research funding decisions are made." This is probably the least-understood aspect of NIH operations and is closely tied to the equally complex budgeting process that determines (subject to OMB and congressional approval) how much funding each institute, program, and mechanism receives.

Each of the 21 separate institutes and centers has its own legislative history, mandate, and budget from Congress, and each differs from the others with respect to its goals, scope, absolute size, and allocation of funding between extramural and intramural research. This highly decentralized and complex structure for the administration and conduct of research has both strengths and weaknesses. Although this diversity has contributed to a research establishment of great vitality and research productivity, it has led to an administrative structure that prevents uniform oversight and planning, hinders coordination of programs that involve several or all of the institutes, and obscures public comprehension. For example, from the short descriptions that each institute and center provided, the committee saw substantial differences in their priority-setting processes, such as the extent to which and how they involve outside groups.

In recent years, the director of NIH has been exercising increased authority to coordinate NIH responses to opportunities and needs that involve multiple institutes. This chapter addresses the adequacy of the priority-setting processes and the analytical and planning capacities needed to coordinate an organization as decentralized as NIH.

The NIH booklet Setting Research Priorities has fairly full discussions of priority-setting criteria and their complexity, descriptions of the various mechanisms used to solicit advice, and lists of the types of individuals, groups, and organizations that are routinely consulted, but it contains little about the planning and budgeting processes that result in the annual budgets and the expanded and new initiatives that those budgets typically contain. The best description was probably provided by NIH Director Harold Varmus to the House appropriations subcommittee in 1997 (U.S. House of Representatives, 1997a:73–76).

In those hearings, the NIH director described priority setting as continuous and occurring at two pivotal levels: at the level of the institute directors and at the level of the director of NIH. The central element of the NIH planning process is the annual meeting of the NIH Leadership Forum, composed of the NIH director, the institute directors, and NIH administrators responsible for major trans-NIH research and management issues (e.g., women's health, rare diseases, and alternative medicine).

PRIORITY SETTING THROUGH THE BUDGET PROCESS

The actual dollar amount allocated to NIH is the result of a complex process of negotiations among OMB, DHHS, the NIH director, and Congress. Because of NIH's commitments to infrastructure and multiyear grants (its commitment base), each year it can realign only a fraction of its budget.[1] More specifically, the NIH director can set new priorities only with additional funds received beyond the commitment base.

Historically, an expansion of research in one area has resulted in a decrease in another area. Only in times of real growth have significant realignments been made. A further constraint on change comes from the fact that each of the institutes receives a separate appropriation from Congress, as do the Office of the Director, the Office of AIDS Research, and buildings and facilities. Budgets are put together from the bottom up (from the institutes and centers and through the NIH director) and are reconciled with budget limits and programmatic priorities imposed at higher levels within NIH, DHHS, and OMB in a long, complex, and interactive process. The institute budget proposals are negotiated with DHHS and OMB through the NIH director, who submits an NIH budget overview to the appropriations committees along with the individual institutes' budgets and, most importantly, works with the appropriations committees on how to distrib-

---

[1]In addition, it is important to note that NIH has several mandated activities requiring collaboration with other federal agencies, such as the Centers for Disease Control and Prevention, the U.S. Food and Drug Administration, the Environmental Protection Agency, the U.S. Department of Defense, and NSF.

ute any budget increases. The director of NIH plays an important role in deciding how much each institute can ask for within the budget total imposed by DHHS and OMB and can, in this way, affect allocations.

Although Congress looks to the director for advice on how to allocate any budget increases that it might give to NIH, the director is limited in this exchange by the requirement to adhere to the budget and priorities set forth by the administration (via NIH negotiations with DHHS and OMB). Thus, the NIH director is unable to communicate directly to Congress, early in the budget process, his or her independent judgment regarding the best use of NIH funds in the coming year.[2] One outcome of this process is that the NIH director at times has been found to be in the position of defending a budget request that is lower than the congressional mark or that reflects priorities that differ from those of Congress and perhaps even those of NIH itself (for example, if a special research directive was issued by DHHS or the White House).[3] Thus, the NIH director probably has the greatest, albeit limited, influence on NIH priority setting during the annual budget process. After the budget is passed, the appropriations are made directly to each institute, which then controls the use of the funds.

Aside from the budget process, which provides little opportunity for radical priority setting, the institutes have two broad opportunities for creating priorities: deciding (1) which grant applications to support through the peer-review process[4] and (2) which research topics to authorize as part of their portfolio. The former opportunity is largely not within each institute's control, whereas the latter is decided through an iterative process involving the NIH director, the institute directors, and the various constituencies served by NIH and its research portfolio. The processes used to accomplish each of those goals are quite different.

---

[2]In contrast, by law, the NCI director can bypass DHHS and OMB in the budget process and go directly to Congress with a budget request that matches directly the professional judgment of NCI and its leadership regarding research needs and priorities. NCI is the only institute with this authority.

[3]For this and other reasons, past reports have recommended that the NIH director report at least to a higher level—to the secretary of DHHS rather than the assistant secretary for health or to the president directly—if not directly to Congress. For example, in 1984 IOM recommended that "the Secretary of Health and Human Services should delegate to the Director of NIH the authority, direction, and control over NIH that the position does not now possess" (Institute of Medicine, 1984).

[4]Peer review is the system used to help decide research funding among competing applications. Although it is not explicitly a system of priority setting, it does rank proposals within a research area in order of scientific impact or significance, which de facto determines the de facto priorities among problems and approaches in that area. The proposals are referred to an institute for funding, and the institute's national advisory council may fund lower-ranked proposals that would have greater relevance to the institute's mission. The NIH peer-review system is under extensive review and is not addressed further in this report.

NIH DIRECTOR'S ROLE IN PRIORITY SETTING

The relative authority of the NIH director has long been a subject of debate and discussion, with many analysts calling for greater influence and centralization. In 1984 IOM wrote, "the Office of the Director is the logical locus for a central coordination activity at NIH" (Institute of Medicine, 1984). Historically, the authority of the director has been limited largely by the size and complexity of the NIH organization and by its budget process. More recently, in 1991, the director's authority was expanded in two specific areas: (1) the director was given the ability to transfer up to 1 percent of funds across institute lines, and (2) the director was given a discretionary fund with which to seed selected areas of research.[5] In addition, the director has played a more active role in priority setting by requiring the institute directors to receive part of their budget increases through an initiative called the NIH Areas of Research Emphasis (described below).

With a unique NIH-wide perspective and ultimate responsibility, the NIH director looks at each institute's programs "with particular emphasis on needs and opportunities for crosscutting efforts" (U.S. House of Representatives, 1997a:73–76). The director accomplishes this through a system of regular senior staff meetings with deputy directors for intramural and extramural research and associate directors for science policy, legislative affairs, and communications and through feedback from interest groups and briefing sessions with institute directors. In addition, the Office of the Director has acquired a number of offices to advise the director of needs and opportunities and to coordinate NIH activities in various areas of concern, for example, rare diseases, alternative medicine, women's health, minority health, and behavioral and social research.

The NIH director oversees 15 offices with a combined budget of $201 million in FY 1998. Roughly one-fourth of this budget supports the operations of the Office of the Director; the remainder supports special functions, such as the Office of Women's Health and the Office of Alternative Medicine. An issue of considerable concern to the Office of the Director in recent years has been the congressional requirement that NIH hold its annual increase in research management and support levels to 1 percent. This has restricted the ability of NIH to engage in more planning and evaluation of programs since those activities are funded through that mechanism.

---

[5]Both authorities were recommended in a 1984 IOM report. In addition, the discretionary fund was recommended in a 1988 IOM analysis, *Report of a Study: A Healthy NIH Intramural Program: Structural Change or Administrative Remedies?* (Institute of Medicine, 1988).

Transfer Authority

The current NIH director has used the transfer authority for the past 3 years as a part of the regular budget process to target specific research opportunities. The NIH director has indicated that he considers other factors as well when making these transfers, such as the effect on new and competing grants, success rates, overall effects on programs "assessed" for transfer funds, and the future impact on programs receiving funds (which will have to absorb the out-year costs).

To receive transfer authority funds, proposals are submitted by institute directors and are reviewed by ad hoc panels of outside reviewers using the criteria of (1) scientific merit and (2) relevance to a broad spectrum of the biomedical research community. In 1995, 1996, and 1997, the NIH director transferred $8.4 million, $24.8 million, and $33.8 million of a possible $110.5 million, respectively. Examples of accomplishments resulting from the receipt of transfer funds include construction of a map of the rat genome; establishment of a national resource for small-angle X-ray scattering and X-ray spectroscopy; establishment of an NIH consortium for research in neurodegenerative and brain disorders; collaborative efforts in programs related to bone, cartilage, and dental diseases; projects in the neurobiology and genetics of autism; and improved preparedness for rapid responses to emerging diseases.

Discretionary Fund

In recent years, the director's power to lead NIH has been strengthened by authorizations for a director's discretionary fund (about $10 million a year). In submitting the NIH budget, the NIH director can identify areas of special emphasis that will receive incentive funding. This approach of providing incentive funding for a focused initiative has stimulated research and fostered collaborations among institutes. Sometimes the research areas are identified at levels above NIH. For example, within the area of the biology of brain disorders, an initiative spurred by the president's commitment to this area was begun in 1997 to encourage research on spinal cord injury. The initiative began with a major workshop that convened experts on spinal cord injury, along with leaders from other scientific areas, to foster new ideas and collaborations. Following the workshop, a program announcement highlighting important relevant research topics was issued. Other funds were used to support such efforts as clinical research training awards, research on an influenza vaccine, genomic research, and an African multilateral initiative on malaria.

NIH Areas of Research Emphasis

In recent years the director has played a more active role in priority setting by requiring the institute directors to receive part of their budget increases through the NIH Areas of Research Emphasis. This initiative has been developed by the current NIH director as a way of planning for and prioritizing the use of funds resulting from the annual incremental budget increases. These Areas of Research Emphasis "provide a broad framework for building new initiatives to confront specific diseases or classes of diseases through laboratory and clinical research" (U.S. Department of Health and Human Services, 1998:5). They typically include research areas that are critical to the scientific agenda of more than one institute and that are fundamentally important to progress in understanding a wide variety of diseases.

The funds available for this initiative can be sizable, depending on the amount of the overall NIH budget increase. For example, the FY 1999 budget increase is more than $1 billion. Of that increase NIH plans to use 52 percent, or $598 million, to support the six Areas of Research Emphasis, including the biology of brain disorders, new approaches to pathogenesis, new preventive strategies against disease, new avenues for the development of therapeutics, genetic medicine, and computers and advanced instrumentation.

These priority initiatives are identified through discussions involving many components of NIH leadership and its stakeholder communities, culminating in a dialogue between the NIH director and each institute or center director. The funds that are allocated through this process become part of the budget base of each institute that receives them. This process has thus become an innovative and influential means of setting research priorities across NIH.

Advisory Committee to the Director

In 1965 a presidentially appointed committee studied NIH and made a series of recommendations, one of which was for a policy council in the director's office:

> A new advisory group should be established to assist the Office of the Director of NIH in the making of major plans and policies, especially those related to the allocation of NIH funds and resources. Referred to as the "Policy and Planning Council," the new unit should consist of experienced and distinguished scientists together with a suitable minority of outstanding non-scientists with wise understanding of and dedication to fulfillment of the Nation's needs (White House, 1965).[6]

---

[6]The report went on to say that the council should not only be called on by the director of NIH "but it should be encouraged by the congressional committees concerned with NIH to participate in the annual budgetary hearings and in the formulation of the NIH programs."

The Advisory Committee to the Director (ACD) was established in 1966 to advise the director and the secretary of the U.S. Department of Health, Education, and Welfare (now DHHS) on NIH policy matters and to make recommendations regarding program development, resource allocation, policies, and regulations. The ACD is chaired by the secretary or the secretary's designee and is chartered to have 16 members: 11 researchers from the private sector and academic research communities and 5 representatives of the public. The President's Biomedical Research Panel recommended in 1976 that ACD be reorganized and strengthened as the NIH Advisory Board, and the IOM committee on the organization of NIH also recommended in 1984 greater use of ACD, stating:

> The current Director's Advisory Committee should be converted to a stronger and more independent NIH Policy and Planning Council to provide for the Director a continuous evaluation of the research mission and function of NIH, and to advise the Director in the formulation of long-term plans and in setting research priorities (Institute of Medicine, 1984:5).

Each NIH director uses ACD in different ways and to various degrees. The NIH director can also use ACD to form special expert panels to provide advice on crosscutting issues. Recent examples include ad hoc panels on gene therapy, clinical research support, human embryo research, the NIH intramural research program, and the peer-review system. Although over the past three decades several committees have recommended that the NIH director use ACD in a more proactive and evaluative way, it is not clear that this has been the case.

PRIORITY SETTING AT THE INSTITUTE LEVEL

Although the NIH director can influence priority setting through participation in the annual budget process, the use of blue ribbon panels to recommend new or reorganized programs, and the use of budgetary authority to launch crosscutting areas of research emphasis, the levels of funding for most of the budget, and therefore the research allocations, are determined at the institute level. NIH is a very large, complex, and decentralized enterprise in which most programming and budgeting activities come from the bottom up.

During its deliberations, the IOM committee received descriptions of each institute's priority-setting process. They reveal widely varying priority-setting processes. Some such variation is appropriate, because the institutes vary in their missions, histories, leadership, sizes, and complexities. Some institutes have more formalized planning and budgeting processes, which tend to be more easily understood by (i.e., transparent to) external constituencies. Some institutes routinely incorporate a wider range of external views, including the views of patients and their advocates.

Some institutes, such as the National Eye Institute, have a long-standing formal planning process for setting priorities. Others, such as NCI, have engaged in an elaborate set of activities to review its programs and progress and have expanded input from consumer advocates. For example, NCI relies on advisory committees (called working groups or review groups) in its priority-setting and planning process, with a mix of members including intramural and extramural researchers, NCI and other federal officials, consumer and patient advocates, and representatives of professional societies and organizations. Still others employ rigorous and well-structured internal and external planning reviews. For example, to review its priorities the National Institute of Allergy and Infectious Diseases (NIAID) engages in twice-annual retreats involving representatives of the scientific community and the public (see Box 3-1 for an example).

BOX 3-1 The Priority-Setting Process at NIAID

The National Institute of Allergy and Infectious Diseases (NIAID) planning process is organized around two major, institute-wide planning meetings that engage the institute director, scientific program head, and senior management staff in a collective effort to identify and establish priorities for future research. The process is designed in sequence with the federal budget formulation process and is thus focused 2 years into the future.

The first step in the process is the Summer Policy Retreat, which provides a forum for planning future scientific directions, for example, tuberculosis research, development of a malaria research strategy, impact of managed care on NIAID research, and human immunodeficiency virus vaccine research. Discussions from this retreat are then transmitted to the NIAID Advisory Council for feedback and input.

A Winter Program review is then convened to consider the deliberations that have preceded it and to define current gaps in knowledge, emerging public health needs, and research opportunities. Specific initiatives are then ranked within a budget projection. Following the Winter Program review, divisions of NIAID submit their proposed initiatives to the budget office. The institute director, in consultation with senior management, then selects the initiatives that will become part of the budget submission to the NIH director. These plans are also submitted to the NIAID Advisory Council for review.

Throughout the process, the institute director and the division directors meet with national organizations, voluntary health organizations, and professional societies. Focus groups are convened at scientific and professional society meetings to receive further input. Input from patient groups occurs at the community level through patient participation on local and national advisory boards that have been established to provide advice to large clinical trials networks.

Each institute also has a national advisory council, the makeup of which is usually determined in the enabling language that created the institute. The national advisory councils review and approve all grants and provide policy advice to the institute director. In most cases, there are 18 members: 12 scientists, chosen for their research expertise, and 6 nonscientists (usually physicians and other professionals rather than representatives of patient groups or groups with special health problems).

Each institute also has a Board of Scientific Counselors, which provides advice on and reviews the intramural research program, and a Board of Scientific Advisors, which provides advice on the extramural programs. Institute directors often form working groups and ad hoc panels to help them address key issues in their research programs. Many institutes have offices for consumer issues. The institutes frequently engage in program reviews or progress reviews to determine if the institute is investing in the appropriate areas of research. NIH has 141 chartered advisory committees (see Appendix A) and makes use of numerous ad hoc advisory committees.

In summary, the institutes have varied systems for receiving advice, planning, and setting priorities. However, there is tremendous variability in the levels of diversity and activism of these activities and in the specificities, scopes, and time frames of the plans developed. For example, some institutes appear to adopt plans developed by a proactive staff with the endorsement of advisory groups, whereas others follow closely the recommendations of external advisory groups.

CONCLUSIONS AND RECOMMENDATIONS

Priority setting is decentralized at NIH, which is appropriate for a research organization in which those closest to a problem are in the best position to decide on approaches and in which expertise is highly specialized. The priority-setting processes also vary from institute to institute and from area to area within institutes. Some such variation is appropriate, because the institutes vary in their missions, histories, leadership, sizes, and complexities. The committee did find that some institutes and programs have priority-setting processes that incorporate a broader range of inputs and views, including those of nonresearchers and nonclinicians.

More recently, NIH has been making decisions on priorities and funding allocations that are more centralized than in the past; that is, NIH is looking across traditionally independent institutes and centers and focusing on certain crosscutting needs and opportunities where joint or unified action is desirable. This trend stems from the growing realization that common biological processes underlie diseases that were previously seen as different or that important diseases and other health problems are more complex than was previously thought, affect more organs and processes than was previously realized, and happen to be addressed in more than one institute.

The committee concluded that the Office of the Director of NIH needs an increased capacity to analyze such crosscutting needs and opportunities and to interact with the public (the latter process-related issue is addressed separately in Chapter 4). Improvement requires a more central role for the NIH director and more uniformity in the data and analyses presented to the Office of the Director.

> ***Recommendation 5.*** **In exercising the overall authority to oversee and coordinate the priority-setting process, the NIH director should receive from the directors of all of the institutes and centers multiyear strategic plans, including budget scenarios, in a standard format on an annual basis.**

In any organization, change toward centralization raises concerns about accountability. As the authority of the director is strengthened, greater accountability of the Office of the Director could be achieved through a strengthened ACD, one that is more actively engaged in the NIH priority-setting process.

> ***Recommendation 6.*** **The director of NIH should increase the involvement of the Advisory Committee to the Director in the priority-setting process. The diversity of the committee's membership should be increased, particularly with respect to its public members.**

The charter of the current ACD gives it this responsibility. However, it meets infrequently and provides advice on matters that do not appear to be sufficient to fulfill this responsibility. Furthermore, although 5 of the 16 ACD slots are for nonscientists with "wise understanding of and dedication to fulfillment of the Nation's needs" (White House, 1965), a review of ACD membership reveals that these reserved slots are not being filled with enough public members consisting of individuals from organized voluntary groups, individuals active in advocating for those with specific diseases or medical conditions, and members of organizations and individuals who represent population groups with special or disproportionate health problems. Not having more public members from these groups is a missed opportunity and has resulted in the perception of some groups that NIH does not encourage public input at the highest levels. The committee recommends that the director of NIH work more actively with the secretary of DHHS in appointing public members to ACD and in providing guidance to ACD on how it can work more effectively in an advisory capacity.

4

Mechanisms for Public Input

Public input is an essential and integral part of any democratic process. Done well, it can improve the knowledge base for decisions, clarify the nature and extent of agreements and disagreements (e.g., among participants and between participants and agencies), and yield more widely accepted decisions (National Research Council, 1989, 1996). In the case of NIH, public participation can help leaders better understand the public's view of health research issues and help citizens better understand critical research policy issues.

Clearly, the public is intensely interested in health, particularly in diseases that affect them personally or those close to them. There is broad agreement among the public, the U.S. Congress, and the executive branch that investing in biomedical research is the right thing to do. Based on the record thus far, Americans hold high expectations for the future achievements of biomedical science, which will provide the return on that investment.

Beyond that apparent consensus, however, are deeply held and sometimes divisive convictions about how research dollars should be spent. Advocates for cancer patients want resources devoted to cancer prevention and treatment just as strongly as advocates focused on effective therapies for diabetes, stroke, or arthritis, for example, or improved research and therapeutic interventions for underserved portions of the population want resources devoted to those causes. With limited funds for health research, various disease-specific interest groups sometimes find themselves at odds with NIH or with each other about the relative size and dimension of the biomedical research portfolio and how it should be apportioned. In some cases, more than one advocacy group might be formed around a given disease, for example, diabetes, Lyme disease, or AIDS. These groups do not always agree on the best research approach to better health. In some cases they may even be diametrically opposed on any given issue. At other times, diverse groups unite on issues of common interest, such as more overall funds for research or reduced regulatory constraints on the conduct of research.

PUBLIC INPUT INTO PRIORITY SETTING

Advocacy is an important and vital part of the biomedical research environment. Disease-specific interest groups have long been a valuable source of support for NIH and its budget (Strickland, 1972). In many ways, advocacy efforts such as those that began in the late 1960s created the modern NIH. When NIH's budget began to stagnate after 1966 (it actually fell for several years), a coalition of disease-specific interest groups and clinical researchers led by Mary Lasker and Sidney Farber mobilized to push through greatly expanded powers and budgets for NCI as part of a "War on Cancer" (Rettig, 1977). After 1970, NIH's budget began to grow again (doubling by 1980 and doubling again by 1990), and the number of research grants went up accordingly. At the same time, disease-specific interest groups, working through Congress, became much more involved in organizational and budget allocation decision making. As a result, the number of institutes increased by seven and the share of funding aimed at specific diseases (as distinct from funding for undirected basic research) grew as other groups sought to achieve the levels of funding achieved by the National Cancer Program.

Advocacy on behalf of health research needs reflects representative democracy and a sense of the public good. It has also shaped NIH's priorities in a way that can be hard to follow or that can lead to abrupt changes in funding patterns—changes that vary in how well they fulfill NIH's own criteria for setting priorities. In addition, specific advocacy efforts can succeed in gaining large increases in funding for certain diseases (e.g., AIDS and breast cancer) at the expense of funding for others.[1] This is especially true when the overall NIH budget has been level or growing slowly.

Thus, in addition to advancing the nation's overall investment in health research, advocacy efforts can create a contentious environment for those trying to set research priorities, be it Congress or NIH. Moreover, interest groups have often produced extensive data sets on disease-specific research spending in an

[1]In 1993, for example, NCI allocations for breast cancer research increased by $53 million, cervical cancer research funding increased by $10 million, ovarian cancer research funding increased by $6 million, and prostate cancer research funding increased by $7 million. To achieve these increases, NCI had to cut basic research funding for leukemia, non-Hodgkin's lymphoma, and cancers of the colon, bladder, kidney, and brain, as well as for public information and chemoprevention (Stephens, 1993).

effort to make the case that too little money is being spent on a given disease, that too much is being spent on another, or that the emphasis of research on a given disease is inappropriate or unbalanced.[2] However, as discussed in Chapter 2, NIH's own criteria for setting priorities recognize that there is no simple metric that can be used to guide how allocations should be set. (Recommendations on better data collection and presentation were presented earlier in this report.)

When a disease-specific interest group believes that insufficient resources are being devoted to its cause, that research emphases are inappropriate, or that there is no mechanism by which it can have input in the priority-setting process, it has two possible courses of action. First, interest groups representing various factions of the public can approach Congress in an attempt to achieve their goals and objectives. Members of Congress have the prerogative of selecting the interests that they wish to serve. In the past, lobbying of members of Congress has been an effective mechanism for disease-specific interest groups. There is no reason to expect that this strategy will not continue to be an effective and legitimate mechanism for public input into the process.

The second course is to approach NIH directly, seeking additional or redirected resources for research important to the group. As with Congress, NIH's responsiveness to interest groups has varied. As a result, some groups feel that their concerns are being heard, whereas others believe either (1) that they cannot gain access to NIH leaders or (2) that when they do gain access, they are met with resistance. To some extent, these variations in perception might be attributable to personalities, differences in leadership, and inconsistent messages on the part of both the interest groups and NIH. In some instances, the perceived lack of responsiveness by NIH to interest group requests is attributable to authentic voids in scientific opportunity or limited resources. In some cases, NIH may simply be unresponsive.

RECENT CHANGES

In recent years, several events have changed the environment in which Congress, NIH, and interest groups interact.

First, in 1994, congressional leadership changed for the first time in nearly four decades. Thus, the leadership and staffing of congressional NIH authorization and appropriations committees changed. Well-established alliances and

---

[2]For example, at the public hearing on April 3, 1998, advocates made various points about research emphases. A representative from the American Heart Association talked about the need for greater emphasis on prevention and compliance research. A representative from the National Alliance for the Mentally Ill asked for a greater focus on biological research and suggested that much of the behavioral research at the National Institute of Mental Health did not reflect patients' priorities.

negotiating tactics were, in some cases, eliminated. Further, in recent years some congressional leaders have called for a cessation in the earmarking of funds for specific diseases. This has frustrated some disease-specific interest groups, who find themselves operating in an environment where the rules have changed; that is, the door appears to have closed before they were able to get inside. Others feel that they have never been able to get their foot in the door.

Second, a new NIH director was appointed in 1993. His immediate goal was to shore up the scientific quality of the nation's biomedical research establishment, because for several years prior to his appointment there had been growing concern that the quality and innovativeness of NIH had sagged (Cohen, 1993a,b; Nature, 1993). The new director adopted a more centralized approach to managing the many institutes and other organizational entities that constitute NIH, and he used new authorities granted the director by Congress to set priorities. This management style had been recommended by numerous advisory groups convened over the past 20 years (Institute of Medicine, 1988; Klausner, 1992; National Institutes of Health, 1994a; U.S. Department of Health, Education, and Welfare, 1976).

Although most observers agree that vesting the director with more authority has been a positive change, it has also placed the current director's office more in the spotlight, resulting in the perception that he should be better able to consider and respond to public input than previous directors.

Third, for some time representatives of some disease-specific interest groups had worked together to seek increased overall funding for NIH, the proverbial "rising tide that lifts all the boats." In the meantime, certain disease-specific interest groups—notably, advocates for AIDS and breast cancer research—were extremely successful in achieving large increases in the NIH budget for research in those areas. This apparent success led other groups to pursue the same tactics to receive equitable funding for their causes. There has also been growth in the use of professional lobbyists, many of them former congressional staff members, by voluntary groups to make their case in Congress. Together, these trends have fueled the perception of some that at times NIH funds research on diseases with the most active groups behind them rather than those diseases for which the needs are greatest in terms of suffering and cost or diseases for which scientific opportunities are the greatest.

In 1997 the Congressional Research Service described the perception of some members of Congress and the public that NIH spending often follows current politics and political correctness or responds to media attention to certain diseases which results in unacceptable disparities in spending. For example, the Parkinson's Action Network claimed that in 1994 NIH spent more than $1,000 per affected person on AIDS research, $93 on heart disease, and $26 on Parkinson's disease. The American Heart Association contended that while overall NIH funding has increased 36 percent in constant dollars since 1986, funding for the heart disease research program at NIH has declined 5.5 percent.

The Juvenile Diabetes Foundation asserted that funding at the National Institute of Diabetes and Digestive and Kidney Diseases increased only 53 percent over a 10-year period when overall NIH funding increased 97 percent (Johnson, 1998).

Finally, some interest groups that have always felt disenfranchised from the biomedical research enterprise continued to feel that their concerns were not being met.

Thus, in the process of setting priorities, Congress and NIH have received input from a large and diverse, although by no means comprehensive, group of organizations and interest groups. Recent disagreements between NIH and these groups over priorities may be due in part to substantive differences in opinion or limitations in the mechanisms for these opinions to be heard and considered by NIH. Although some mechanisms for public input, both formal and informal, currently exist, sufficiently recognizable and accessible points of entry do not exist for those who wish to provide public input but who are unfamiliar with the intricacies of NIH's current complex and varied priority-setting processes. This flaw has exacerbated long-term, unresolved issues about the relative influence of disease-specific interest groups on the NIH priority-setting process. It has also contributed to newer and more acute issues raised by the changes in the environment in which disease-specific interest groups and members of Congress are now operating. It is clear that broader involvement of the public in discussions about NIH priority setting can result in positive outcomes by enhancing the relevancy of research programs, improving the design and conduct of research, particularly patient-oriented studies, and assuring all those with an interest in NIH research that there is an opportunity to be heard.

TWO-WAY COMMUNICATION BETWEEN NIH AND THE PUBLIC

In addition to conducting and supporting research and training to improve health, NIH has a major responsibility for informing the public about biomedical research and for responding to the views of various publics on research priorities. An important part of this responsibility is the communication or dissemination of research results and health information, which, done well, involves active outreach to and involvement of the public in planning and evaluation. The committee was not, however, in a position to evaluate NIH's performance in these areas, its use of current communications or education research, or the quality of its own evaluations. Instead, it focused on the public role in the research priority-setting process at NIH. Specifically, the committee reviewed the "transparency" of the priority-setting process—that is, making clear how NIH makes decisions and allocates resources, how interested citizens may become involved in programs of interest to them, and how public interests are incorporated in NIH's external advisory system.

For example, one function that does not seem to have been addressed very fully is explaining the mission and workings of NIH and, especially, how it sets priorities. NIH's recent booklet "Setting Research Priorities at the National Institutes of Health" (National Institutes of Health, 1997b) describes the system, but the explanation is complicated and does not indicate how concerned people can provide input to the priority-setting process, especially those who would not naturally have easy access to this process.

NIH interacts with various constituencies, including

- extramural research scientists,
- non-research-oriented clinicians who apply research results and who can identify research needs (physicians, including specialized physicians, nurses, dentists, pharmacists, social workers, psychologists, public health practitioners, and other allied health practitioners),
- organized voluntary groups and individuals active in advocating for those with specific diseases or medical conditions, and
- organizations and individuals who represent population groups with special or disproportionate health problems (members of particular ethnic groups, low-income populations, women, elderly people, children, etc.).

The institutes and centers have different priority-setting processes, that is, they differ in how they plan research programs and allocate resources among them, and they also differ in the extent and nature of public involvement in their advisory systems. Where to go to find out about NIH's programs or to express interests and concerns would not always be obvious to an interested individual or group. The situation is further complicated when an issue involves multiple institutes, and the Office of the Director is not always equipped to handle public input about issues that cut across NIH or involve several institutes.

NIH has long-standing mechanisms by which to include public or lay members on top-level advisory bodies. In most institutes, for example, 6 of 18 membership slots of the national advisory council are reserved for public representatives. These councils provide to the institutes advice and guidance on their research programs and funding decisions by providing the second layer of review (the first being peer review through the study sections). Thus, public representatives play a role in the priority-setting process and provide advice on funding decisions. Review of the memberships of these councils reveals that some institutes do not appear to be filling these reserved slots with enough public members representing the last two groups in the list above, that is, representatives of patients and their families and of populations with special health problems. Not doing so is a missed opportunity and has resulted in the perception of some groups that NIH does not encourage public input at the highest levels of its advisory processes.

Each institute also has a National Council or a Board of Scientific Counselors, which provides advice on and reviews the intramural research program, and a Board of Scientific Advisors, which provides advice on the extramural programs. (Appendix A lists the advisory boards for each institute.) In addition, institute directors often form working groups and ad hoc panels to address key issues in their research programs. Institutes frequently engage in program or progress reviews to determine whether the institute is investing in the appropriate areas of research. Some institutes have offices for consumer and public issues (see Box 4-1 for a description of the NCI Director's Consumer Liaison Group as an example of an exemplary public advisory body at NCI).

BOX 4-1 The NCI Director's Consumer Liaison Group

The NCI Director's Consumer Liaison Group was formed to help NCI develop mechanisms to increase the level of representation of the cancer advocacy community on NCI advisory committees and to increase consumer-advocate involvement in NCI's program and policy development (National Cancer Institute, 1997). To form the Director's Consumer Liaison Group, a consultant was hired and charged with the responsibility of contacting individual scientists, health care provider organizations, disease-specific interest groups, community-based organizations, and minority and nonminority science organizations and soliciting nominations.

Eligibility requirements included the following:

- A "public individual" who has experience with either a specific disease or disabling condition or with disease prevention and health maintenance, for example, a disease-specific interest group, a person affected by the consequences of a disease or disability, a professional or volunteer who works with survivors or those affected, or a member of community-based organization dealing with health issues of a particular community.
- Someone who represents a constituency (formally or informally) with which she or he regularly communicates on issues pertaining to clinical care or research and who is able to serve as a conduit for information both to and from his or her constituency.
- Someone with a commitment to working with NIH on issues relevant to care for people with a particular disease or disabling condition and research on a disease or disability.

In addition, ACD of NIH reserves 5 of its 16 slots for public members. Unlike the national councils at each institute, ACD does not oversee or advise the director on a specific research portfolio, except for whatever advice it provides on the use of the director's discretionary funds, transfer authority, or Areas of Research Emphasis (see Chapter 3). Presumably, the NIH director may consult with ACD on the overall NIH budget or new initiatives as he or she sees fit. As with the national councils at each institute, it appears that the "public" slots of ACD are sometimes not filled by individuals one would commonly consider to represent the public. It is recognized that identifying individuals who can broadly represent the public's interest is a difficult task, but it is nonetheless a worthy goal to be pursued because of the importance of a public presence on the advisory committee closest to the director of NIH. The committee believes that priority setting at NIH would be improved and its outcomes would be better understood and accepted if advisory bodies had more consumers and advocates from among all of the categories of constituencies listed above.

Although many of the institutes primarily rely on scientists and health professionals for external advice, the committee encountered a number of examples in which institutes and offices have incorporated a broader range of external inputs, including the involvement of patients and their advocates, in their priority-setting processes. For example, in addition to NCI's consumer liaison group, it also invites advocates and consumer groups to sit on panels reviewing organizational and disease-specific components of its research program, such as, cancer centers or progress in prostate cancer research. NIAID has a broad-based formal planning process that is not only transparent (that is, clearly described in documents and charts) but that also involves a range of public viewpoints, including those of patients and advocates who participate in planning retreats and other forums. NIAID has also established the extensive use of community advisory boards in its clinical trials, cohort studies, and other clinical research groups "to bring about greater involvement of community advocates and potential [clinical] trial participants in scientific and protocol planning . . . and provide a forum for concerns that may arise among trial participants and the local community" (National Institutes of Health, 1998d:10). The National Institute on Aging developed a book on exercise for older people after receiving numerous inquiries from the public and is working with the Alliance on Aging Research in disseminating the book to the public and health care providers (National Institutes of Health, 1998d:14). The Office of AIDS Research holds an annual planning workshop that includes nongovernment experts and AIDS community representatives. The NIH AIDS research program recently underwent a thorough evaluation by a group of scientists and community activists. That study, which also relied on the findings of a series of review panels consisting of scientists from industry and academia and community advocates, resulted in a number of major changes. The report of the NIH AIDS Research Program Evaluation Working Group describes the process and lists the participants (National Institutes of Health, 1996). The National Institute of Environmental Health Sciences and the Office of Minority Health have each held town meetings around the country to increase public understanding of NIH programs and solicit public input.

CONCLUSIONS AND RECOMMENDATIONS

Given the changes in the environment in which Congress, NIH, and the interest groups are now operating, NIH faces a special challenge to better interact with the public, receive public input, and demonstrate that such input is fully considered, even though it is not necessarily adopted. To this end, the committee recommends three approaches to improving NIH's interface with the public. The committee reached these recommendations after concluding that NIH, especially the Office of the Director, does not have adequate channels through which the public can provide broad input into the NIH priority-setting process or through which NIH can respond clearly and authoritatively to the public on issues of mutual concern.

The committee based its conclusions on several findings. First, patient advocacy groups have become better organized and more proactive on behalf of their interests and have greatly increased their appeals to Congress to intervene to adjust NIH research priorities. Second, congressional leaders have expressed a strong desire to avoid mandates and earmarks in favor of particular diseases and to let NIH set research priorities. Third, the NIH director has increased his role in priority setting (partly by exercising additional authorities granted to him by Congress), but a formal mechanism through which the public can inform the priority-setting process is lacking. This confluence of events highlights the need for improved communication between the public and NIH.

The following recommendations are not intended to replace the existing criteria for priority setting. They are intended to provide new mechanisms or reinforce existing NIH mechanisms through which public voices can be heard in a constructive and open manner. The committee believes that public input, which has been important in sustaining the growth and stature of NIH, is an essential component of the priority-setting process and if used wisely will make for a stronger and more responsive NIH. It also recognizes that although these recommendations, if implemented, will improve the priority-setting process at NIH, they will not supersede or remove the potential for alternative approaches to public input, such as appeals to Congress.

NIH should engage the public to a greater extent in informing the process by which NIH sets its research priorities. The following three recommendations are intended to provide the public with more opportunities to present their views regarding research needs and to receive information about research and the priority-setting process at NIH.

> ***Recommendation 7.*** **NIH should establish an Office of Public Liaison in the Office of the Director and, where offices performing such a function are not already in place, in each institute. These offices should document, in a standard format, their public outreach, input, and response mechanisms. The director's Office of Public Li-**

aison should review and evaluate these mechanisms and identify best practices.

Recommendation 8. **The director of NIH should establish and appropriately staff a Director's Council of Public Representatives, chaired by the NIH director, to facilitate interactions between NIH and the general public.**

Recommendation 9. **The public membership of NIH policy and program advisory groups should be selected to represent a broad range of public constituencies.**

Offices of Public Liaison: Rationale, Roles, and Responsibilities

Establishing an Office of Public Liaison within the Office of the NIH Director will facilitate and enhance two-way communication with the public and go far toward addressing the concerns of Congress and the public about how NIH sets research priorities. As a staff operation, the key functions of the Office of Public Liaison should include the following:

1. Receiving input from a broader range of constituencies, disease-specific interest groups, and those concerned about underserved or underrepresented populations that are (or that have the potential to be) interested in the prioritization and results of NIH research. Although no parallel structure is in place to represent various scientific interest groups, the committee believes that effective mechanisms to represent those interests are already in place.
2. Organizing this input in a way that can be informative in priority setting.
3. Documenting the ways in which input is provided to those involved with NIH decision-making processes and NIH's responses to this input.
4. Involving NIH leadership in receiving and responding to input from the public.
5. Advising the Office of Communications so that NIH maximizes its resources by providing information and programs that are most responsive to the public.
6. Evaluating the activities listed above.

In addition, because public input can be directed either to the Office of the Director or to a specific institute, it is important that each institute have an office or officer responsible for public liaison. The existence of such staff offices in each institute—with a common and understandable name or title—will provide a visible place for the public to go when seeking input or information. The key functions of each institute's Office of Public Liaison would be similar to those of the Director's Office of Public Liaison. In addition, because it is routine for the Office of the Director to refer "institute-specific" inquiries to the appropriate institute (e.g., a question about research programs related to prostate cancer would be referred to NCI), the establishment of such offices in each institute and in the Office of the Director would create a coordinated network similar to that which already exists among the offices of communication and the offices of legislative affairs. The Offices of Public Liaison at each institute would routinely report to and meet with the staff of the Director's Office of Public Liaison to share information and develop policy. Through this system each institute director would be served, as would the NIH director.

In summary, the Offices of Public Liaison serve several purposes: (1) they provide an easily identifiable point of contact for individuals and groups who have an interest or concern; (2) they are a place where Congress can refer constituents; and (3) they conduct an active program of outreach to and interaction with constituency groups. The Offices of Public Liaison would be staff offices and thus would function every day, unlike advisory groups, and most of their effort would be to provide information to and receive input from interested groups and congressional offices.

The committee recognizes that the Offices of Public Liaison might impose additional costs and complicate organizational coordination. However, most institutes already have staff who perform many of the functions, so the net additional cost would not be as large as it might seem. For some of the smaller institutes, the Office of Public Liaison function could probably be performed by one individual. The more complex organizational issue will be to work out clear relationships among Offices of Public Liaison and existing offices of communication and legislative affairs.

Given the importance of the public outreach function in NIH's overall mission, especially after it is expanded and reorganized in accord with this recommendation, the director of NIH should consider putting this set of functions of the Office of Public Liaison under an associate director who is on the same functional level as the other associate directors in the Office of the Director.

It is also imperative that additional funds and personnel be made available to fulfill the goals of public liaison. Current restrictions on the research management and support budget should be adjusted or the research management and support budget should be increased to accommodate these recommendations. The extra personnel needed to staff the Offices of Public Liaison should be considered exempt if the limits on research management and support persist (see also Recommendation 12 in Chapter 5).

Across NIH, the new Offices of Public Liaison would also establish initiatives aimed at reaching out to special populations that would not normally have easy access to these communications processes. Precisely how this realignment of functions would entail the reorganization of current offices of communication, which are responsible for the dissemination of research results and for patient and provider education, would be left to each institute, depending on its missions and how it is currently organized. Institutes should identify educational, communications, and outreach needs through appropriate research and should pre- and posttest their materials and processes for their effectiveness.

The NIH director's Office of Public Liaison should coordinate the development, testing, and dissemination of outreach materials. In addition, staff in the director's Office of Public Liaison should routinely collect from the 21 institutes and centers data relevant to each institute's responsibilities, report their findings to the NIH director, and respond to requests from interest groups that cannot be adequately referred to appropriate institutes and centers or whose interests cross multiple institutes. The director's Office of Public Liaison should ensure that there is an open flow of information among NIH staff and between NIH staff and interest groups (including congressional staff). The staff of the director's Office of Public Liaison would coordinate activities with parallel offices in each of the institutes and centers and with the director's Office of Communications and Office of Legislative Policy and provide staffing for the Director's Council of Public Representatives.

Director's Council of Public Representatives: Rationale, Roles, and Responsibilities

The recommendation to create a Director's Council of Public Representatives is aimed at addressing a major weakness: the lack of a forum for the director of NIH to interact constructively and in a systematic and regular way with representatives of the public. Clearly, disease-specific interest groups are seeking access to the NIH director in record numbers, especially given the recent reluctance of Congress to respond to their concerns via the earmarking of funds. If the NIH director were to meet personally with each of these groups, he or she would have little time for anything else. Yet, there should be a systematic and well-planned mechanism by which interest groups can have access to the Office of the Director, if not the director personally. Although each institute has its own disease-specific constituencies, particularly the categorical, disease-centered institutes, some interest groups can find no logical home in the NIH federation or find that many institutes conduct research relevant to their interests but that there is no clear lead institute. In addition, when an interest group believes that its needs are not being met at the institute level, that group might identify the Office of the Director as the logical place to register its concerns.

The proposed Council is distinct from the Offices of Public Liaison, which are identifiable staff offices that provide full-time points of contact and channels of communication with interested individuals and groups about NIH priorities and programs. Moreover, the Offices of Public Liaison do not provide a mechanism for the direct interaction of the public with the NIH director, as does the Council. It is the committee's view that the establishment of a Council elevates the importance of public input in informing the process by which NIH sets its research priorities and provides a more feasible mechanism by which the NIH director can receive and respond to such public input. Currently, the director receives such input on an ad hoc basis and meets with groups independently. The proposed new Council offers an organized, regular mechanism for the director to obtain consumer views by providing an opportunity for various interests to interact directly with the NIH director on issues of mutual concern, discuss the priority-setting process, and suggest constructive measures to improve public input and participation. In addition to substance, establishment of the Council has the advantage of being highly visible and a symbol of NIH's concern about the views of those affected by the health problems that are the focus of NIH-funded research—patients, their families, and those who advocate for them. The committee believes that it would go a long way toward reducing the pressure on Congress to micromanage NIH as well as serving as a valuable forum in which the director and public representatives can share their views and concerns.

As an advisory council, the key functions would be to interact on a formal basis three to four times a year and advise the NIH director on how best to

- develop potential mechanisms for interaction with and engagement of the public in the NIH priority-setting process, including the review of the activities of the Offices of Public Liaison;
- achieve broad representation of the public on standing and ad hoc policy and program advisory bodies, including national advisory councils;
- enhance public understanding of the mission and priority-setting process of NIH;
- consider the health concerns of special populations, for example, members of particular ethnic groups, underserved individuals, elderly people, women, children, and those with chronic diseases or disabling conditions;
- refine and improve the presentation of data on the allocation of research funds for particular diseases;
- identify best practices for receiving public input and advocating their replication across NIH; and
- identify and recruit public members for participation across NIH.

Importantly, the Director's Council will not set priorities regarding the NIH budget or its research programs. That is, it is not intended to serve as a forum for advocacy groups to lobby the NIH director for research dollars. Rather it is intended to serve as a mechanism for NIH to receive valuable and thoughtful perspectives on its research programs from those who are in some way affected by disease and disability and who are therefore advocates for a healthy NIH, and to provide information about its research and priority-setting process as part of a two-way exchange of information.

The Director's Council of Public Representatives should be made up of 18 to 25 individuals representing a broad range of public constituencies of NIH (e.g., disease-specific interest groups, ethnic groups, public health advocates, and health care providers). They should be appointed for staggered 3-year terms. The Director's Council of Public Representatives should be chaired by the NIH director and should be staffed by the director's Office of Public Liaison (obviating the need for additional staff to support the Council).

The Council should issue an annual report evaluating the progress of public input and activities and whether this input and these activities have had specific effects on the NIH research program. The main potential drawbacks of the Council would be the raised expectations that would result from its establishment and the difficulties of appointing a representative group from among hundreds of constituencies. NIH will have to state and constantly restate that public input is one source of information about public health needs, that public health needs is one criterion among many considered in setting research priorities, and that in any case, the Council is not charged with making decisions about NIH's priorities, only with informing the process. Thus, although the Council will not be able to satisfy all interest groups with the outcomes of NIH's actions, it will increase the chances that all concerned will judge the process to be a fair one in which various views receive a respectful airing and a thoughtful response. Over time, the Council's activities will help to create a common frame of reference through which interest groups and scientists can obtain an understanding of and can articulate their concerns and constraints. Figure 4-1 shows the proposed placement of the Offices of Public Liaison and the Director's Council of Public Representatives within the current organization at NIH.

Policy and Program Advisory Group Membership

The committee also believes that the NIH priority-setting process would be improved if broader representation were extended to all policy and program advisory bodies at NIH, such as standing and ad hoc advisory groups on programs and research agendas within and across institutes. By this, the committee recommends that NIH use its existing capacity to include public representatives on standing advisory committees (through already mandated reserved seats for public members) and through enhanced public input where appropriate. NCI, NIAID, the National Institute of Environmental Health Sciences, and other institutes, centers, and offices provide good examples, in that they have in place processes and structures for effectively involving consumers in priority setting, policy and program advisory bodies, and the annual budgeting process. The Director's Council of Public Representatives, recommended above, could play a role in identifying best practices and advocating their replication across NIH. In addition, an important responsibility of the Council will be to help identify and recruit public members for participation across NIH.

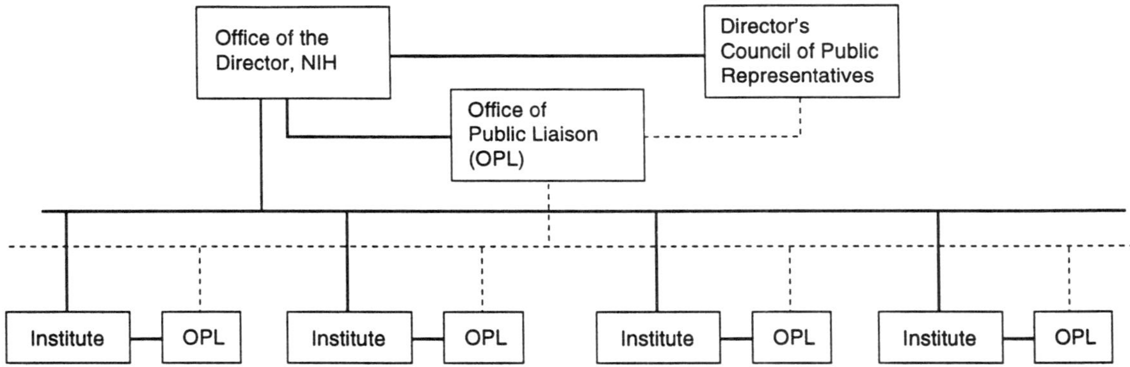

FIGURE 4-1 Proposed placement of the Offices of Public Liaison and the Director's Council of Public Representatives within the current organization at NIH.

Each institute should aim for public participation that is sufficiently broad, that uses a selection process that is fair and that is perceived to be fair, and that incorporates representatives participants from disease-specific and other interest groups and who bring to the process the kind of knowledge, experience, and perspectives that are needed for the deliberation at hand.

Summary

The new organizational mechanisms for improving public input proposed here have the potential to increase, in the short term, organizational costs and complexity. In the long run, however, the committee believes that the contribution made by these offices and the Council will prove to be cost-effective in terms of carrying out NIH's mission to improve health through research and will contribute to overall goodwill on the part of the public and Congress toward NIH. Each entity—the Director's Council of Public Representatives, the network of Offices of Public Liaison, and the existing advisory bodies to the director of NIH and the institutes—has its own rationale and roles that should improve NIH's priority-setting process.

5

Congressional Role

The fourth charge to the committee was to "assess the impact of statutory directives on research funding decisions." The committee broadened the charge to address the role of Congress in setting NIH research priorities through various means, including the use of report language, which is often used instead of statutory language to communicate congressional priorities to NIH.

CONGRESS AND NIH

The members of Congress who serve on one of the four main committees affecting NIH—the House and Senate authorization subcommittees and the House and Senate appropriations subcommittees—are more familiar with how science works than Congress as a whole and are aware of the problems caused by earmarking or other overprescriptive directives that reduce NIH's flexibility to set priorities informed by scientific opportunity as well as need. The health committees have been less prescriptive in recent years, but those who want Congress to specify funding of research on particular diseases can go, and recently have gone, to other places in the system. In recent years, for example, there have been earmarks for breast cancer research and prostate cancer research in defense legislation and an appropriation for diabetes research in the Balanced Budget Act.

Legislators on the NIH-related subcommittees also often have their own ideas about how NIH might better carry out its mission. Some become interested for one reason or another in a particular disease or medical condition. Some become interested in the health of particular groups, such as women, members of minority groups, elderly people, and children. Some worry that NIH is not paying enough attention to or investing adequately in particular kinds of research—the state of clinical research is currently a big issue—or crosscutting activities (such as prevention or nutrition) or important fields, technologies, and approaches (such as bioengineering, medical imaging, and alternative medicine).

For these reasons, authorization bills and appropriations committee reports have until recently contained some fairly specific directives. These have included mandates to establish particular offices or centers in institutes or in the Office of the Director, the use of certain mechanisms (such as centers, clinical trials, or specific requests for applications), or the use of set-asides of specified amounts of funding for a particular activity.

Many Congressional leaders would prefer to rely on NIH to allocate funds among research programs, but first, they are mindful of their important oversight responsibility. NIH is part of a very important public function and has a very large budget. Second, members of Congress are constantly approached by individuals and groups about the impacts of terrible diseases, and they want to show that they are trying to help. At the same time, many believe that NIH should be making the decisions about the allocation of funding among research areas, because they are aware that the opportunity for advances varies from one problem to another. Thus, the legislators want to be able to refer people to an identifiable process at NIH and be assured that NIH is in fact listening and taking what they hear into account, that is, that the inputs of all interests have been fairly and appropriately taken into account in program and resource allocation decision making.

The existence of such a process is not clear to all members. Members of Congress are constantly exposed to disease-specific interest groups that have statistics on disease burdens and lists of scientific opportunities and argue that they are neglected in terms of the amount of funding for research on their disease of interest as reported by NIH. They wonder: How does NIH know that an area of research is emerging and when and how to respond? How are measures of disease burden and costs taken into account and how does the public have input? Does the NIH priority-setting process need to be changed, or is it working well and the need is just for better communication?

How Congress Communicates Priorities

As noted, NIH operations, structure, and funding are affected most by four congressional committees: the authorization and appropriations committees in each house. The authorization committees are the House Committee on Commerce (Subcommittee on Health and Environment) and the Senate Committee on Labor and Human Resources (Subcommittee on Public Health and Safety).

The appropriations committees are the House Appropriations Committee (Subcommittee on Labor, Health and Human Services, and Education) and the Senate Appropriations Committee (Subcommittee on Labor, Health and Human Services, and Education).

Appropriations Process

Historically, the appropriations committees have played a major role in NIH priority setting. They usually appropriate millions more than the president's budget requests, which makes it much easier to influence, if not specify, the use of the appropriation than is the case with appropriations for other agencies in which Congress appropriates about the same amount or a little more or less than the amount requested by the administration.

Appropriations committees have a number of ways of communicating intent about executive agency priority setting, including bill language, report language, statements made on the House or Senate floor or at hearings, and informal contacts between committee members and staff and agency officials. All these methods are used in the case of NIH.

Statutory Language The language used in NIH appropriations laws is usually general. Typically they read: "for carrying out section 301 and title IV of the Public Health Service Act with respect to cancer [or diabetes and digestive and kidney diseases, or allergy and infectious diseases, etc.], $*x*." However, statutory language is always an available route if Congress feels strongly about something and NIH has not responded to concerns expressed in report language.

For example, in the first session of the 105th Congress, Congress took the unusual step of including as an amendment to the FY 1998 appropriations bill a revision of the Public Health Service (PHS) Act of 1944 that authorized a program of research on a specific disease, Parkinson's disease (the Udall Bill). Although the appropriations committees did not give the amendment a specific appropriation, the National Institute of Neurological Disorders and Stroke is responding using the basic authority contained in the PHS Act (section 301). In November 1997, it issued an RFA for Parkinson's Disease Research Centers of Excellence.

Report Language Report language is the normal means of expressing congressional intent. Although directives in report language do not have the force of law, NIH takes them quite seriously. For one thing, if NIH does not respond, the directive could escalate into statutory language in a subsequent session of Congress. For another, for both Congress and NIH report language is a more flexible means of communication than bill language. The problem for NIH comes when the language is too detailed and ends up forcing NIH to fund more research than there are good projects to support or to use particular mechanisms.

Examination of the FY 1993 and FY 1998 reports of the appropriations committees reveals examples of many kinds of directives, ranging from "the Committee is encouraged by the Institute's continued support of research on *x*" to "the Committee has provided $25 million for *y* disease research, $4 million more than requested and $5 million more than last year's level." The typical item in report language "encourages" or "urges" that NIH or the institute continue to make *x* a high priority or to expand support. There are many types of directives, however. The list includes the following:

- Specify a dollar amount for a particular program (Office of Alternative Medicine) or particular area of research (e.g., pediatric research initiative or Alzheimer's disease).
- Specify a mechanism, for example, saying that the committee has put in sufficient funds (or a specific funding amount) to support a new research center or a specific number of research centers addressing a particular disease, that NIH should issue an RFA, or that NIH should begin planning clinical trials.
- Call for a scientific conference on opportunities in a particular field or disease to be held and a report submitted before the next year's appropriations hearings.
- Require that a formal report be made on a topic of interest. This is partly done to express interest in that topic and is often done to look for suggestions for research opportunities that Congress can urge NIH to fund (if Congress has not done so already).
- Ask for a 5- or 10-year research plan to be submitted to the committee by a certain date and require consultation with the affected outside groups.
- Ask the NIH director to assign a clear lead agency (e.g., NIAID and Lyme disease in the FY 1993 Senate report).
- Suggest that NIH consider setting up a separate study section for a disease on which the committee wants to see more emphasis.
- Suggest a type of national advisory council member (the Senate committee suggested, for example, that the National Eye Institute add an optometrist).
- Direct that an intramural program be expanded or formalized.

The typical directive—"the Committee encourages the institute to expand its support of *x* research"—is usually not problematic because, given NIH's normal rate of budget growth, research on *x* is going to grow anyway, without any special steps being taken. In many cases, the institute can simply document in its next year's congressional justification budget and in testimony what would have happened anyway. That is not always the case, however. In the late 1980s and early 1990s, NIH budget growth slowed and the number of earmarks specifying amounts of spending on particular disease programs grew. The earmarks sometimes added up to more than the budget increases, and so some institutes had to find ways to pay for them, which in turned squeezed other programs. In FY 1993, for example, the appropriations committees earmarked additional funding for research on breast, ovarian, cervical, and prostate cancers that was more than the total increase of $28 million that they gave to NCI for cancer research. The earmarks added up to $77 million, which NCI offset by cutting basic research and research on leukemia; non-Hodgkin's lymphoma; cancers of the colon, bladder, kidney, and brain; public information and education; and chemoprevention. Other examples include an earmark of $24 million for pediatric AIDS clinical trials in the FY 1991 House report. In that case, the conference committee agreed on a final overall amount for NIAID that was $34 million less than the House recommendation but specifically directed that the increase for pediatric AIDS clinical trials stay at $24 million, which resulted in cuts in vaccine development and other areas of AIDS research.

Trends in Appropriations Reports The numbers of items in the reports accompanying the appropriations bills increased between the reports for the 2 years that the committee examined in detail (1993 and 1998), but the items included far fewer earmarks for specific levels of funding for particular programs or other detailed directives in the latter year (see Table 5-1). The Senate, for example, specified $133 million in FY 1998, whereas it specified $785 million in FY 1993.

TABLE 5-1 Numbers of Significant Items in Reports Accompanying Appropriations Bills, FY 1993 and 1998

Report	FY 1993	FY 1998
House Appropriations Report	115	150
Senate Appropriations Report	193	201

Authorization Process

Historically, NIH has benefited from having a permanent authorization (section 301 of the PHS Act of 1944 gives the secretary of DHHS broad permanent authority to conduct and sponsor research) and from the practice, begun in 1948, of authorizing "such sums as may be necessary." Historically, the main action in the authorization process was whether or not to create new institutes. The pressures that this puts on Congress resulted in the 1984 study by an IOM committee of the organizational structure of NIH (Institute of Medicine, 1984).

Since then the number of institutes and other major units (centers and divisions) has increased to 21. Beginning with the example of the AIDS research buildup in the 1980s, the focus among disease-specific interest groups has shifted to tracking the amount of funding across NIH for their particular interest and trying to impose more crosscutting coordination of programs, for example, by establishing a tracking and coordinating office in the Office of the Director of NIH.

The 1993 Reauthorization The most recent reauthorization was in 1993, and a reiteration of its provisions indicates the trends (U.S. Congress, 1993):

- Reauthorized certain expiring authorities of NIH.
- Mandated establishment of the Office of Research Integrity in DHHS.
- Lifted the moratorium on human fetal tissue transplantation research.
- Mandated inclusion of women and minorities in clinical research protocols.
- Established the Office of Alternative Medicine in the Office of the Director.
- Established the Office of Research on Women's Health in the Office of the Director.
- Established the Office of Biobehavioral and Social Sciences Research in the Office of the Director.
- Put the National Center for Human Genome Research on a statutory basis.
- Mandated establishment of an intramural laboratory and clinical research program on obstetrics and gynecology within the National Institute of Child Health and Human Development (NICHD).
- Established the National Center on Sleep Disorders Research in the National Heart, Lung, and Blood Institute (NHLBI).
- Codified in statute the establishment of the Office of AIDS Research and strengthened and expanded its authorities, including the authority to receive all AIDS appropriations and disburse them to the institutes and centers.
- Authorized establishment of an NIH director's discretionary fund.
- Provided the NIH director with extramural construction funds (with a set-aside of $5 million for centers of excellence).
- Mandated establishment of the Institutional Development Award Program.
- Required NCI to conduct the Long Island breast cancer study.
- Authorized scholarship and loan repayment programs for individuals from disadvantaged backgrounds.
- Elevated the nursing center to an institute, the National Institute for Nursing Research.
- Elevated the NHLBI Division of Blood Research to a center.
- Provided a number of other new NIH authorities and directives.

The 1996 Senate Reauthorization Bill The Senate (but not the House) passed a reauthorization bill in 1996. The pressure to mandate programs and organizational units for particular purposes was intense. The subcommittee tried to avoid specificity. According to its report on the NIH Revitalization Act of 1996 (U.S. Senate, 1996):

> In crafting this legislation, the committee wrestled with the question: Should the Congress be directive and authorize more set-asides for specific diseases, or should it authorize institute funding that enables scientific discovery itself to determine the directions for research funding? In general, the committee tends toward the view that the latter is the better course to make resources available to scientists to pursue new knowledge where it leads. The committee believes that this strategy has been highly productive in the NIH assault on the diseases that afflict Americans.

Despite the subcommittee's intentions, the report and accompanying bill in fact contained a number of new set-asides and other provisions that affected NIH priority setting by mandating programs for and directing resources toward specific diseases. Most of them were added as amendments. The bill did the following:

- Elevated the genome center to institute status, the National Human Genome Research Institute, and mandated a set-aside of at least 5 percent of the new institute's extramural research funds for research on ethical, legal, and social issues.
- Included provisions intended to increase support for clinical or patient-focused research by NIH.
- Established a Parkinson's disease research and training program with up to 10 core grants for Morris K. Udall Centers for Research on Parkinson's disease, with \$80 million authorized for the first year and such sums as may be necessary for the next 2 years (added by amendment).
- Increased the authorization for diabetes research by 25 percent over the next 3 years (added by amendment).
- Created an office of pediatric research in the Office of the Director "to increase pediatric biomedical research," with increased funding to be allocated by the director after consultation with external advisers and NICHD (the bill authorized \$50 million a year for the next 3 years) (added by amendment).
- Required NIH to report how it is going to implement an earlier report to Congress, Support for Bioengineering Research.
- Codified the Office of Rare Disease in the director's office.
- "Encouraged" the NIH director to establish a Pain Research Consortium involving all NIH units involved in pain research (in lieu of an amendment to establish a National Center for Pain Research at NIH and six regional centers for pain research).

Current Situation Some committee members (e.g., Senator Dan Coats [U.S. Congress, 1997b]) expressed strong reservations about the wisdom of legislating in such detail. One result was the series of hearings that the Senate subcommittee held on priority setting at NIH, beginning on May 1, 1997, in an effort to reach an understanding among members of Congress and between Congress and NIH on the desirability of letting NIH decide on most if not all allocations below the institute level (see discussion in Chapter 1).

Although most witnesses in the May 1, 1997, hearing on NIH priority setting and several that followed favored letting NIH set priorities and opposed detailed directives from Congress, the authorization committees face intense pressures to use the reauthorization bill to accomplish specific goals. Current proposals include

- a Center for Alternative Medicine,
- codification of the General Clinical Research Centers in the PHS Act,
- a new Institute on Biomedical Imaging,
- a Center on Bioengineering in NHLBI,
- a pediatrics initiative,
- a proposal to use $2.5 billion from a tobacco settlement and earmark one-third for behavioral research, and
- initiatives left over from the 1996 reauthorization, including the National Center for Pain Research and a diabetes program.

CONCLUSIONS AND RECOMMENDATIONS

The U.S. Congress has always played an active role in setting research priorities at NIH. For example, it periodically decides to create new institutes or other organizational entities and routinely allocates funds among NIH institutes and centers and other units through the annual appropriations process. It may mandate the amount of spending or specify mechanisms of research on particular areas or diseases (e.g., mandating the establishment of centers or the issuance of RFAs) if it concludes that NIH is neglecting opportunities or needs.

Congress, of course, has the authority, which it has felt compelled to use from time to time, to intervene in NIH's affairs, for example, by mandating the creation of a center or office or by specifying a funding level for research on a particular disease. The committee agrees, however, with the sentiments of many legislators that Congress should rely as much as possible on NIH's own priority-setting processes because Congress generally lacks the expertise to judge the degree of scientific opportunity. The committee believes that implementation of its recommendations would go a long way toward ensuring a process that interest groups will find to be open and fair and, hence, would reduce the level of public appeals to Congress.

It appears to the committee that in general the Congress has eased up on its use of earmarks and other restrictive directives in recent years. Although the number of congressional directives has increased, they are much less specific. For example, the number of earmarks for funding for research related to particular diseases has declined significantly. Congress's use of report language to convey concerns and priorities is positive, but the specification of budget amounts or specific mechanisms for funding (e.g., mandating that a certain number of centers be established or that a specific RFA be issued) should be done only as a last resort, because these approaches often have unintended effects. For example, in testimony to the committee, an advocate for AIDS research reported that earmarked funds, provided in response to the requests of advocates, had had unexpected negative impacts on other, at least equally important areas of AIDS research. Earmarking of funds for specific diseases also pits disease-specific interest groups against one another.

As science changes, however, and new health problems emerge, NIH must shift its priorities and make organizational changes to adapt. Such changes are taking place all the time. The establishment of the Center for Human Genome Research and its later elevation to institute status are examples. The creation of the Office of AIDS Research is another example. In these and other cases, if commitments of substantial new funding or major organizational changes are involved, Congress invariably becomes involved through the reauthorization process. Groups and organizations that believe that their interests will be helped by the creation of a new NIH unit (by increasing visibility and funding) will ask Congress to authorize such funding. Indeed, as mentioned above, there are a number of current proposals to mandate new organizational entities and levels of funding for specific diseases in pending NIH reauthorization legislation.

What guidelines can the committee offer Congress to help it determine whether to specify a new program, center, or institute? In 1984, an IOM committee recommended criteria to be used to evaluate proposals for new institutes or other major organizational changes (see Box 5-1).

Perhaps more importantly, the 1984 IOM committee also recommended that NIH rely on a range of activities short of establishing new institutes to respond to health needs and opportunities. That committee suggested that NIH have "a continuum of possible responses to needs and opportunities it identifies, matched with the magnitude and urgency of the demand" (Institute of Medicine, 1984:19):

> • publicizing what scientific research has accomplished, and the status and promise of current research in the area;
>
> • disseminating the results of research widely to centers that can make immediate clinical use of them;
>
> • accelerating research by such means as soliciting applications for grants, scheduling special peer review sessions, appointing special study sections, and utilizing "high relevance scores" for applications in the area concerned;
>
> • holding major conferences with the leaders among the scientists and practitioners concerned to exchange ideas and discuss future actions and, in

appropriate situations, creating such groups by action of the Secretary of Health and Human Services, or the White House, or by joint action with Congress;

- naming special panels or subcommittees of the national advisory councils, boards of scientific counselors, review committees, and study sections, as appropriate, to examine both extramural and intramural programs and opportunities;
- forming an NIH-wide or interagency committee, preferably led by an institute director, to coordinate and develop research in the area; and
- providing higher visibility and stronger leadership over the area of concern by organizational upgrading; for example, elevating sections to branches, branches to programs, or programs to divisions.

BOX 5-1 Criteria for Organizational Change

To focus the debate about the costs and benefits of new institutes, the committee recommends that the following five criteria be considered in evaluating proposals for organizational change:

1. The activity of a new institute or other organizational entity must be compatible with the research and research training mission of NIH. If a major emphasis of the proposed new entity is regulation, the delivery of services, or other non-research-related activities, it is not appropriate for incorporation into NIH.
2. It must be demonstrable that the research area of a new institute or other major organizational entity (defined either as a disease or health problem or as a biomedical or behavioral process related to a health problem) is not already receiving adequate or appropriate attention.
3. There must be reasonable prospects for scientific growth in a research area to justify the investment in a new institute or other major organizational entity.
4. There must be reasonable prospects of sufficient funding for a new institute or other major organizational entity.
5. A proposed change in the NIH organizational structure should, on balance, improve communication, management, priority setting, and accountability.

SOURCE: Institute of Medicine (1984:21–23).

The situation has changed since 1984. There are still calls for new institutes and centers. Today, however, the main focus of interested groups is on having Congress mandate NIH-wide programs or funding levels, or both, for specific diseases or other activities.

The present committee finds that the approach of the 1984 committee is still a good one. However, it sees the need to elaborate it to address other demands or responses beyond the creation of new NIH organizational entities. Additional responses that NIH could take short of congressional action include inclusion of an area in the NIH Director's Areas of Research Emphasis, designation of lead institutes, and establishment of a coordinating office in the Office of the Director of NIH.

> ***Recommendation 10.*** **The U.S. Congress should use its authority to mandate specific research programs, establish levels of funding for them, and implement new organizational entities only when other approaches have proven inadequate. NIH should provide Congress with analyses of how NIH is responding to requests for such major changes and whether these requests can be addressed within existing mechanisms.**

NIH has an obligation to engage in periodic reviews of its organizational structure and planning and budgeting systems and to explain the results to Congress and the public, if it is to manage its own priority setting rather than react to directives from Congress trying to respond to requests from disease-specific interest groups. Such reviews would result in NIH making organizational and management changes, including the creation or disestablishment of institutes and centers and the reorganization of existing ones, or requesting new or expanded authorities from Congress, when needed. The reviews should also include evaluations of past organizational and management changes to see if they have been successful. This flexibility would help NIH remain organizationally dynamic and would help it incorporate changing scientific knowledge and meet health needs in a well-considered and planned way.

> ***Recommendation 11.*** **The director of NIH should periodically review and report on the organizational structure of NIH, in light of changes in science and the health needs of the public.**

Through the appropriations process, Congress directed NIH to reduce the budget for research management and support by 7.5 percent in FY 1996 and did not allow increases in FY 1997 or FY 1998 (although activities designated as related to public health education were exempted from the cap in FY 1998). Those cuts came after reductions had already been made in response to the administration's Reinventing Government initiative.

Congress's intent was to reduce administrative overhead. However, as NIH is currently organized, research management and support includes a number of important program-related functions. It includes, for example, the personnel and other expenses (e.g., travel) of reviewing extramural research proposals and managing the grants that are subsequently funded by NIH (it does not include the intramural research program). The extramural grant program is the largest and fastest-growing part of NIH's research effort. Research management and support also includes the capacities that need to be expanded to improve research priority-setting activities at NIH, such as new or expanded Offices of Public Liaison, the new Director's Council of Public Representatives in the Office of the Director, increased consumer participation in all NIH advisory bodies, and improved collection and analysis of disease-related data.

Resources invested in these underfunded functions not only should help NIH to fulfill its mission of improving the nation's health but should also improve the effectiveness of public oversight of its activities, thus enabling Congress and interest groups to observe and participate in a process that is more transparent and more satisfactory. This in turn may catalyze a change in which NIH and the consumers of health research work together rather than against each other and in which Congress lets NIH (informed by stronger public input) set research priorities.

> ***Recommendation 12.*** **Congress should adjust the levels of funding for research management and support so that NIH can implement improvements in the priority-setting process, including stronger analytical, planning, and public interface capacities.**

Any additional resources needed to implement this recommendation do not necessarily have to affect the total amount appropriated to NIH. The recommendation is meant to affect the cap on research management and support funding within NIH budgets, if Congress elects to impose caps in future appropriations as it has in recent years.

References

Agnew, B. 1996. Body-Count Budgeting: New Pressure to Shift Funding Among Diseases. Journal of NIH Research June 1996:21–22.

Biotechnology Industry Organization. 1998. 1997–98 BIO's Citizens' Guide to Biotechnology [WWW document]. URL http://www.bio.org/whatis/citizen1.dgw (accessed June 18, 1998).

Cohen, J. 1993a. Conflicting Agendas Shape NIH. Science 261:1674–1679.

Cohen, J. 1993b. Is NIH's Crown Jewel Losing Luster? Science 261:1120–1127.

Institute of Medicine. 1976. The Current Burden of Illness in the United States. Washington, D.C.: National Academy Press.

Institute of Medicine. 1984. Responding to Health Needs and Scientific Opportunity: The Organizational Structure of the National Institutes of Health. Washington, D.C.: National Academy Press.

Institute of Medicine. 1988. Report of a Study: A Healthy NIH Intramural Program: Structural Change or Administrative Remedies? Washington, D.C.: National Academy Press.

Institute of Medicine. 1990. Funding Health Services Research: A Strategy to Restore Balance. Washington, D.C.: National Academy Press.

Institute of Medicine. 1991. The AIDS Research Program of the National Institutes of Health. Washington, D.C.: National Academy Press.

Institute of Medicine. 1994. Careers in Clinical Research: Obstacles and Opportunities. Washington, D.C.: National Academy Press.

Institute of Medicine. 1997. Enabling America. Washington, D.C.: National Academy Press.

Johnson, J. A. 1998. Disease Funding and NIH Priority Setting. CRS Report for Congress. Report 97-917 STM. Washington, D.C.: Congressional Research Service.

Klausner, R. D. 1992. Report of the Task Force on the Intramural Research Program of the National Institutes of Health. Bethesda, Md.: National Institute of Child Health and Human Development.

McGinnis, J. M., and W. H. Foege. 1993. Actual Causes of Death in the United States. Journal of the American Medical Association 270:2207–2212.

National Institutes of Health. 1994a. Report of the External Advisory Committee of the Director's Advisory Committee, The Intramural Research Program, National Institutes of Health. Bethesda, Md.: National Institutes of Health.

National Institutes of Health. 1994b. Section 1125, NIH Organization and Functions. *In* NIH Manual. Bethesda, Md.: National Institutes of Health (revised October 1, 1994).

National Institutes of Health. 1996. Report of the NIH AIDS Research Program Evaluation Working Group of the OARAC. Bethesda, Md.: National Institutes of Health.

National Institutes of Health. 1997a. Disease-Specific Estimates of Direct and Indirect Costs of Illness and NIH Support, 1997 Update. Bethesda, Md.: National Institutes of Health.

National Institutes of Health. 1997b. Setting Research Priorities at the National Institutes of Health. Bethesda, Md.: National Institutes of Health.

National Institutes of Health. 1997c. Review Criteria for and Rating of Unsolicited Research Grant and Other Applications. NIH Guide 26:22.

National Institutes of Health. 1997d. NIH Organization Handbook. Bethesda, Md.: National Institutes of Health.

National Institutes of Health. 1998a. Press Release for the President's FY 1999 Budget for the National Institutes of Health, February 2. Bethesda, Md.: National Institutes of Health.

National Institutes of Health. 1998b. General Background Information—National Institutes of Health (NIH) [WWW document]. URL http://www.nih.gov/welcome/nihnew.html (accessed May 13, 1998).

National Institutes of Health. 1998c. The President's Fiscal Year 1999 NIH Budget Summary, February 2, 1998 [WWW document]. URL http://www.nih.gov/news/Budget99/BUDGET99.HTM (accessed May 13, 1998).

National Institutes of Health. 1998d. Examples of How Research Priorities Have Been Affected by Public Input. Provided to the Committee on the NIH Research Priority-Setting Process by the Office of Science Policy, NIH, April 2. Bethesda, Md.: National Institutes of Health.

National Research Council. 1989. Improving Risk Communication. Washington, D.C.: National Academy Press.

National Research Council. 1996. Understanding Risk. Washington, D.C.: National Academy Press.

National Science Foundation. 1997a. Federal R&D Funding by Budget Function, Fiscal Years 1994–1996. NSF 97-301. Arlington, Va.: National Science Foundation.

National Science Foundation. 1997b. Federal Funds for Research and Development, Fiscal Years 1995, 1996, and 1997, Vol. 45, Detailed Statistical Tables. NSF 97-327. Arlington, Va.: National Science Foundation.

Nature. 1993. NIH: A Strategy for the 21st Century? Nature 363:99–100.

NIH Director's Panel on Clinical Research. 1997. Report to the Advisory Committee to the NIH Director. Bethesda, Md.: NIH Director's Panel on Clinical Research.

Office of Management and Budget. 1997. Instructions for the Preparation and Submission of Annual Budget Estimates. Circular A-11. Washington, D.C.: Office of Management and Budget.

Pharmaceutical Research and Manufacturers of America. 1997. 1997 Industry Profile. Washington, D.C.: Pharmaceutical Research and Manufacturers of America.

Rettig, R. A. 1977. Cancer Crusade: The Story of the National Cancer Act of 1971. Princeton, N.J.: Princeton University Press.

Stephens, M. 1993. Testimony before the President's Cancer Panel, Special Commission on Breast Cancer. Reston, Va. July 21.

Strickland, S. P. 1972. Politics, Science, and Dread Disease: A Short History of United States Medical Research Policy. Cambridge, Mass.: Harvard University Press.

U.S. Congress. 1993. Conference Committee Report Accompanying NIH Reauthorization Act of 1993. Washington, D.C.: U.S. Government Printing Office.

U.S. Congress. 1997a. P.L. 105-78, Sec. 213. U.S. Departments of Labor, Health and Human Services, and Education Appropriations Act of 1998. Washington, D.C.: U.S. Government Printing Office.

U.S. Congress. 1997b. Congressional Record, September 3, 1997. Washington, D.C.: U.S. Government Printing Office.

U.S. Department of Health, Education, and Welfare. 1976. Report of the President's Biomedical Research Panel. DHEW Publication No. (OS) 76-500. Washington, D.C.: U.S. Department of Health, Education, and Welfare.

U.S. Department of Health and Human Services. 1998. Justification of Estimates for Appropriations Committees, FY 1999, NIH, Vol. V, Office of the Director. Washington, D.C.: U.S. Department of Health and Human Services.

U.S. House of Representatives. 1997a. Departments of Labor, Health and Human Services, Education, and Related Agencies Appropriations for 1998, Hearings before the Subcommittee on the Departments of Labor, Health and Human Services, Education, and Related Agencies, House Committee on Appropriations. Washington, D.C.: U.S. Government Printing Office.

U.S. House of Representatives. 1997b. Overview of NIH Programs, Hearing before Subcommittee on Health and Environment of the House Committee on Commerce. Serial No. 105-43. Washington, D.C.: U.S. Government Printing Office.

U.S. Senate. 1996. Report Accompanying S. 1897, NIH Revitalization Act of 1996. Washington, D.C.: U.S. Government Printing Office.

U.S. Senate. 1997a. Biomedical Research Priorities: Who Should Decide? Senate Hearing 105-68. Washington, D.C.: U.S. Government Printing Office.

U.S. Senate. 1997b. Coordination of NIH Research Efforts: Three Case Studies. Senate Hearing 105-188. Washington, D.C.: U.S. Government Printing Office.

U.S. Senate. 1997c. Support Strategies for Clinical Research and Alternative Medicine at the NIH. Senate Hearing 105-246. Washington, D.C.: U.S. Government Printing Office.

Varmus, H. 1997. Interview with Harold Varmus. Journal of NIH Research 9(8):21–25.

White House. 1965. Biomedical Science and Its Administration: A Study of the National Institutes of Health. Washington, D.C.: White House.

Wingo, P. A., L. A. G. Ries, H. M. Rosenberg, D. S. Miller, and B. K. Edwards. 1998. Cancer Incidence and Mortality, 1973–1995. Cancer (Cancer Cytopathology) 82:1197–1207.

Appendixes

A

Federal Advisory Committees of the National Institutes of Health

OFFICE OF THE DIRECTOR

Advisory Committee to the Director, National Institutes of Health (NIH)
Advisory Committee on Research on Minority Health
Advisory Committee on Research on Women's Health*
Alternative Medicine Program Advisory Council*
Office of AIDS Research Advisory Council*
Peer Review Oversight Group
Recombinant DNA Advisory Committee
Special Programs Emphasis Panel of the Office of the Director, NIH

NATIONAL CANCER INSTITUTE

Advisory Committee to the Director, National Cancer Institute
National Cancer Advisory Board*
Acrylonitrile Study Advisory Panel
Board of Scientific Counselors, National Cancer Institute
Frederick Cancer Research and Development Center Advisory Committee
President's Cancer Panel*
National Cancer Institute Board of Scientific Advisors
National Cancer Institute Initial Review Group
National Cancer Institute Special Emphasis Panel

---

*Nondiscretionary (statutory) committees.

NATIONAL EYE INSTITUTE

National Advisory Eye Council*
Board of Scientific Counselors, National Eye Institute
National Eye Institute Special Emphasis Panel

NATIONAL HEART, LUNG, AND BLOOD INSTITUTE

National Heart, Lung, and Blood Advisory Council*
Sickle Cell Disease Advisory Committee
Board of Scientific Counselors of the National Heart, Lung, and Blood Institute
Clinical Trials Review Committee
Heart, Lung, and Blood Program Project Review Committee
Sleep Disorders Research Advisory Board*
National Heart, Lung, and Blood Institute Special Emphasis Panel

NATIONAL HUMAN GENOME RESEARCH INSTITUTE

National Advisory Council for Human Genome Research
Board of Scientific Counselors, National Human Genome Research Institute
Center for Inherited Disease Research Access Review Committee
National Human Genome Research Institute Initial Review Group
National Human Genome Research Institute Special Emphasis Panel

NATIONAL INSTITUTE ON AGING

National Advisory Council on Aging*
Task Force on Aging Research*,**
Board of Scientific Counselors, National Institute on Aging
National Institute on Aging Initial Review Group
National Institute on Aging Special Emphasis Panel

NATIONAL INSTITUTE ON ALCOHOL ABUSE AND ALCOHOLISM

National Advisory Council on Alcohol Abuse and Alcoholism*
National Commission on Alcoholism and Other Alcohol-Related Problems*,**

---

*Nondiscretionary (statutory) committees.
**Inactive committees (to be terminated by legislation).

Board of Scientific Counselors, National Institute on Alcohol Abuse and Alcoholism
National Institute on Alcohol Abuse and Alcoholism Initial Review Group
National Institute on Alcohol Abuse and Alcoholism Special Emphasis Panel

NATIONAL INSTITUTE OF ALLERGY AND INFECTIOUS DISEASES

AIDS Research Advisory Committee, National Institute of Allergy and Infectious Diseases *
Board of Scientific Counselors, National Institute of Allergy and Infectious Diseases
National Advisory Allergy and Infectious Diseases Council*
Acquired Immunodeficiency Syndrome Research Review Committee
Allergy, Immunology, and Transplantation Research Committee
Microbiology and Infectious Diseases Research Committee
National Institute of Allergy and Infectious Diseases Special Emphasis Panel

NATIONAL INSTITUTE OF ARTHRITIS AND MUSCULOSKELETAL AND SKIN DISEASES

National Arthritis and Musculoskeletal and Skin Diseases Advisory Council*
National Advisory Board for Arthritis and Musculoskeletal and Skin Diseases*,**
Board of Scientific Counselors, National Institute of Arthritis and Musculoskeletal and Skin Diseases
Arthritis and Musculoskeletal and Skin Diseases Special Grants Review Committee
National Institute of Arthritis and Musculoskeletal and Skin Diseases Special Emphasis Panel

NATIONAL INSTITUTE OF CHILD HEALTH AND HUMAN DEVELOPMENT

National Advisory Child Health and Human Development Council*
National Advisory Board on Medical Rehabilitation Research*

---

*Nondiscretionary (statutory) committees.
**Inactive committees (to be terminated by legislation).

Board of Scientific Counselors, National Institute of Child Health and Human Development
National Institute of Child Health and Human Development Initial Review Group
National Institute of Child Health and Human Development Special Emphasis Panel

NATIONAL INSTITUTE ON DEAFNESS AND OTHER COMMUNICATION DISORDERS

National Deafness and Other Communication Disorders Advisory Council*
National Deafness and Other Communication Disorders Advisory Board*,**
Board of Scientific Counselors, National Institute on Deafness and Other Communication Disorders
Communication Disorders Review Committee
Deafness and Other Communication Disorders Programs Advisory Committee
National Institute on Deafness and Other Communication Disorders Special Emphasis Panel

NATIONAL INSTITUTE OF DENTAL RESEARCH

National Advisory Dental Research Council*
Board of Scientific Counselors, National Institute of Dental Research
National Institute of Dental Research Special Grants Review Committee
National Institute of Dental Research Special Emphasis Panel

NATIONAL INSTITUTE OF DIABETES AND DIGESTIVE AND KIDNEY DISEASES

National Diabetes and Digestive and Kidney Diseases Advisory Council*
National Diabetes Advisory Board*,**
National Digestive Diseases Advisory Board*,**
National Kidney and Urologic Diseases Advisory Board*,**
End-Stage Renal Disease Data Advisory Committee, Health Care Financing Administration / National Institute of Diabetes and Digestive and Kidney Diseases*,**
Board of Scientific Counselors, National Institute of Diabetes and Digestive and Kidney Diseases

---

*Nondiscretionary (statutory) committees.

**Inactive committees (to be terminated by legislation).

Diabetes and Digestive and Kidney Diseases Special Grants Review Committee
National Institute of Diabetes and Digestive and Kidney Diseases Special Emphasis Panel

NATIONAL INSTITUTE ON DRUG ABUSE

Board of Scientific Counselors, National Institute on Drug Abuse
National Advisory Council on Drug Abuse*
National Institute on Drug Abuse Initial Review Group
National Institute on Drug Abuse Special Emphasis Panel

NATIONAL INSTITUTE OF ENVIRONMENTAL HEALTH SCIENCES

National Advisory Environmental Health Sciences Council*
Advisory Council on Hazardous Substances Research and Training*,**
Board of Scientific Counselors, National Institute of Environmental Health Sciences
Environmental Health Sciences Review Committee
National Institute of Environmental Health Sciences Special Emphasis Panel

NATIONAL INSTITUTE OF GENERAL MEDICAL SCIENCES

National Advisory General Medical Sciences Council*
Minority Programs Review Committee
National Institute of General Medical Sciences Initial Review Group
National Institute of General Medical Sciences Special Emphasis Panel

NATIONAL INSTITUTE OF MENTAL HEALTH

National Advisory Mental Health Council*
Board of Scientific Counselors, National Institute of Mental Health
National Institute of Mental Health Initial Review Group
National Institute of Mental Health Special Emphasis Panel

---

*Nondiscretionary (statutory) committees.
**Inactive committees (to be terminated by legislation).

NATIONAL INSTITUTE OF NEUROLOGICAL DISORDERS AND STROKE

National Advisory Neurological Disorders and Stroke Council*
Board of Scientific Counselors, National Institute of Neurological Disorders and Stroke
National Institute of Neurological Disorders and Stroke Initial Review Group
Training Grant and Career Development Review Committee
National Institute of Neurological Disorders and Stroke Special Emphasis Panel

NATIONAL INSTITUTE OF NURSING RESEARCH

National Advisory Council for Nursing Research*
National Institute of Nursing Research Initial Review Group
National Institute of Nursing Research Special Emphasis Panel

NATIONAL LIBRARY OF MEDICINE

Board of Regents of the National Library of Medicine*
Board of Scientific Counselors, National Center for Biotechnology Information, National Library of Medicine
Board of Scientific Counselors, National Library of Medicine
Biomedical Library Review Committee
Literature Selection Technical Review Committee
National Library of Medicine Special Emphasis Panel

WARREN GRANT MAGNUSON CLINICAL CENTER

Board of Governors of the Warren Grant Magnuson Clinical Center
The Board of Scientific Counselors of the Warren Grant Magnuson Clinical Center

JOHN E. FOGARTY INTERNATIONAL CENTER

John E. Fogarty International Center Advisory Board

---

*Nondiscretionary (statutory) committees.

NATIONAL CENTER FOR RESEARCH RESOURCES

National Advisory Research Resources Council*
Scientific and Technical Review Board on Biomedical and Behavioral Research Facilities*,**
National Center for Research Resources Initial Review Group
National Center for Research Resources Special Emphasis Panel

CENTER FOR INFORMATION TECHNOLOGY

Board of Scientific Counselors, Division of Computer Research and Technology

CENTER FOR SCIENTIFIC REVIEW

Center for Scientific Review Advisory Committee
AIDS and Related Research Initial Review Group
Biobehavioral and Social Sciences Initial Review Group
Biochemical Sciences Initial Review Group
Biophysical and Chemical Sciences Initial Review Group
Cardiovascular Sciences Initial Review Group
Cell Development and Function Initial Review Group
Endocrinology and Reproductive Sciences Initial Review Group
Genetic Sciences Initial Review Group
Health Promotion and Disease Prevention Initial Review Group
Immunological Sciences Initial Review Group
Infectious Diseases and Microbiology Initial Review Group
Musculoskeletal and Dental Sciences Initial Review Group
Neurological Sciences Initial Review Group
Nutritional and Metabolic Sciences Initial Review Group
Oncological Sciences Initial Review Group
Pathophysiological Sciences Initial Review Group
Sensory Sciences Initial Review Group
Surgery, Radiology, and Bioengineering Initial Review Group
Behavioral and Neurosciences Special Emphasis Panel
Biological and Physiological Sciences Special Emphasis Panel
Chemistry and Related Sciences Special Emphasis Panel
Clinical Sciences Special Emphasis Panel
Microbiological and Immunological Sciences Special Emphasis Panel
Multidisciplinary Sciences Special Emphasis Panel

---

*Nondiscretionary (statutory) committees.
**Inactive committees (to be terminated by legislation).

B

Acknowledgments

The committee would like to thank all those who took the time to attend and participate in its meetings and share their views with the committee either verbally or as written comments. All of those who participated in panel discussions before the committee, including those at the public meeting, are listed below. A list of those who submitted written comments to the committee follows.

PANELISTS

Norman B. Anderson
Office of Behavioral and Social Research
National Institutes of Health

Stanley Baum
Academy of Radiology Research

Christine Brunswick
National Breast Cancer Coalition

Marvin Cassman
National Institute of General Medical Sciences
National Institutes of Health

Francis S. Collins
National Human Genome Research Institute
National Institutes of Health

Mayer B. Davidson
American Diabetes Association

Morgan Downey
American Obesity Association

Robin Elliott
Parkinson's Disease Foundation

Anthony Fauci
National Institute of Allergy and Infectious Diseases
National Institutes of Health

Annette Ferebee
American Public Health Association

Gregg Gonsalves
Treatment Action Group

David Goodman
National Marfan Foundation

Phillip Gorden
National Institute of Diabetes and Digestive and Kidney Diseases
National Institutes of Health

Enoch Gordis
National Institute on Alcohol Abuse and Alcoholism
National Institutes of Health

Alastair Gordon
The Islet Foundation

Patricia Grady
National Institute of Nursing Research
National Institutes of Health

Laura Lee Hall
National Alliance for the Mentally Ill

William Harlan
Office of Disease Prevention
National Institutes of Health

Robin Harrison
Diabetes Cure Now

Christine Hartel
American Psychological Association

Daniel Hoffman
Association of Schools of Public Health

Steven Hyman
National Institute of Mental Health
National Institutes of Health

David Johnson
Federation of Behavioral, Psychological, and Cognitive Sciences

Karen Johnson
Facioscapulohumeral Dystrophy Society, Inc.

Elke Jordan
National Human Genome Research Institute
National Institutes of Health

Stephen Katz
National Institute of Arthritis and Musculoskeletal and Skin Diseases
National Institutes of Health

Melinda Kelley
Paralyzed Veterans of America

Ruth Kirschstein
National Institutes of Health

Richard Klausner
National Cancer Institute
National Institutes of Health

Michael Langan
Vice President of Public Policy
National Organization for Rare Disorders

Claude Lenfant
National Heart, Lung, and Blood Institute
National Institutes of Health

Robert Levine
Juvenile Diabetes Foundation

Elaine Locke
American College of Obstetricians and Gynecologists

Gina Luke
Association of American Dental Schools

Gerard Lynam
American Diabetes Association

Yvonne T. Maddox
National Institute of Child Health and Human Development
National Institutes of Health

Tony Mazzaschi
Association of American Medical Colleges

Debbie McCoy
Arthritis Foundation

Ray Merenstein
Research!America

Richard A. Millstein
National Institute on Drug Abuse
National Institutes of Health

Jeanette Nottemius
Latino Council on Alcohol and Tobacco

Kenneth Olden
National Institute of Environmental Health Sciences
National Institutes of Health

Daniel Perry
Alliance for Aging Research

Anne Phelps
Legislative Assistant
Office of Senator Bill Frist

Tari G. Radin
Association of Women's Health, Obstetric and Neonatal Nurses

Sandra Raymond
National Osteoporosis Foundation

Michael R. Rosen
American Heart Association

Dom Ruscio
C & R Associates

Peggy Schnoor
Office of Science Policy
National Institutes of Health

Lana Skirboll
Office of Science Policy
National Institutes of Health

Harold C. Slavkin
National Institute of Dental Research
National Institutes of Health

Philip M. Smith
Former Executive Officer
National Research Council

Anne Thomas
Office of Communications
National Institutes of Health

Cheryl Trepagnier
Autism Society of America Foundation

Harold Varmus
Director
National Institutes of Health

Michael Welsh
American Society for Clinical Investigation

Jack Whitescarver
Office of AIDS Research
National Institutes of Health

Vincent W. Yang
American Gastroenterologic Association

WRITTEN COMMENTS

Individuals

Russell V. Boham
Richard R. Clayton
Kelly Ellis-Craig
K. Fischbeck
Boguslaw Lipinski
Daniel Moore
Yufang Shi
Linda Snetselaar
David Spiegel
John K. Wooden
Laurie Worden
Richard Zorowitz

Organizations*

Alzheimer's Association
American Academy of Physical Medicine and Rehabilitation
American Association for Dental Research
American Association for the Surgery of Trauma
American Association of Neurological Surgeons
American College of Rheumatology
American Geriatrics Society
American Society for Microbiology
Center for the Advancement of Health
Congress of Neurological Surgeons
Federation of American Societies for Experimental Biology
National Alliance for Eye and Vision Research
National Council on Family Relations
National Kidney Foundation
Polycystic Kidney Research Foundation
Robert Wood Johnson Foundation
Society for the Advancement of Women's Health Research
Society for the Psychological Study of Social Issues
Summit Health Coalition
Tourette Syndrome Association

INTERVIEWS AND OTHER CONTRIBUTIONS

Margaret Anderson
Society for the Advancement of Women's Health Research

Sarah Brookhart
American Psychological Society

*In addition to those listed under "Panelists."

Miriam Davis
Independent Consultant

Dorothy Foellmer
National Cancer Institute
National Institutes of Health

Ellen Gadbois
Subcommittee on Public Health and Safety
Senate Committee on Labor and Human Resources

Ron Geller
National Heart, Lung, and Blood Institute
National Institutes of Health

Joe Harford
National Cancer Institute
National Institutes of Health

Craig Higgins
National Human Genome Research Institute
National Institutes of Health

Gar Kaganovich
RAND Corporation

Rachel Levinson
Office of Science and Technology Policy
Executive Office of the President

Francine Little
Office of Financial Management
Office of the Director
National Institutes of Health

Anne E. Phelps
Subcommittee on Public Health and Safety
Senate Committee on Labor and Human Resources

Lee Pushkin
Office of Financial Management
Office of the Director
National Institutes of Health

Lana Skirboll
Office of Science Policy
Office of the Director
National Institutes of Health

Michael A. Stephens
Van Scoyic Associates

Irene Stith-Coleman
Congressional Research Service

Anne Thomas
Office of Communications
Office of the Director
National Institutes of Health

Vincent Ventemiglia
Subcommittee on Children and Families
Senate Committee on Labor and Human Resources

Diane Wax
Office of Legislative Policy and Analysis
Office of the Director
National Institutes of Health

C

National Institutes of Health Funding Tables

The acronyms used in these tables are defined in the list of acronyms on p. *xi*.

TABLE C-1 Total NIH Funding by Institute, Center, and Division (in thousands of dollars)

Institute, Center, or Division	FY 1998 Estimate	FY 1999 Estimate
NCI	$2,320,900	$2,536,061
NHLBI	1,522,178	1,646,479
NIDR	195,922	214,559
NIDDK	858,478	927,492
NINDS	754,370	815,649
NIAID	650,186	702,040
NIGMS	1,037,253	1,114,886
NICHD	607,281	654,716
NEI	346,036	374,356
NIEHS	323,556	348,090
NIA	517,369	556,070
NIAMS	270,369	291,053
NIDCD	198,857	213,834
NIMH	649,363	701,790
NIDA	359,777	395,129
NIAAA	212,722	230,243
NINR	58,043	62,416
NHGRI	214,657	236,996
NCRR	371,506	422,995
FIC	17,678	19,105
NLM	157,814	171,253
Office of the Director	201,118	212,949
Buildings and facilities	195,357	218,886
Office of AIDS Research	1,607,053	1,730,796
Total budget authority	13,647,843	14,797,843

SOURCE: National Institutes of Health, FY 1999 President's Budget, 1998, p. 9.

TABLE C-2 Total NIH Funding by Mechanism (in thousands of dollars)

Mechanism	FY 1997 Budget Authority	FY 1998 Estimate	FY 1999 Estimate
Research project grants (RPGs)			
Noncompeting	$4,998,308	$5,487,847	$5,719,127
Administrative supplements	89,123	76,341	82,019
Competing	1,817,248	1,905,898	2,280,898
SBIR/STTR	249,885	262,300	289,462
Total RPGs	7,154,564	7,732,416	8,371,506
Research centers	1,086,282	1,166,974	1,253,450
Other research	583,005	641,140	743,245
Research training	417,087	429,820	510,731
R&D contracts	844,253	880,260	953,601
Intramural research	1,345,287	1,416,161	1,502,359
Research management and support	485,018	493,545	507,832
Cancer control	231,918	254,731	277,707
Construction	22,876	23,000	23,000
National Library of Medicine	150,376	161,185	174,725
Office of the Director	229,717	241,654	254,701
Subtotal	12,550,383	13,440,886	14,572,857
Buildings and facilities	200,000	206,957	224,986
Total budget authority	12,750,383	13,647,843	14,797,843

NOTE: SBIR = Small Business Innovation Research; STTR = Small Business Technology Transfer.

SOURCE: National Institutes of Health, FY 1999 President's Budget, 1998, p. 12.

TABLE C-3 Total NIH Funding for Basic, Applied, and Development Research and Development (in millions of dollars)

Type of Research	FY 1997 Budget Authority	FY 1998 Estimate	FY 1999 Estimate
Basic research	$6,851.4	$7,359.9	$7,976.0
(% of total)	(57.1)	(57.2)	(57.3)
Applied research	3,669.5	3,937.5	4,199.8
(% of total)	(30.6)	(30.6)	(30.2)
Development	1,473.5	1,569.5	1,739.2
(% of total)	(12.3)	(12.2)	(12.5)
Total research	11,994.4	12,866.9	13,915.0
R&D facilities	222.9	229.9	248.0
Training and overhead	533.1	551.0	634.8
Total appropriation	12,750.4	13,647.8	14,797.8

SOURCE: Office of Financial Management, NIH, 1998.

TABLE C-4 Total NIH Funding by Disease or Area of Research (in millions of dollars)

Disease or Area of Research	FY 1997 Budget Authority	FY 1998 Estimate	FY 1999 Estimate
Aging[a]	$978	$1,039	$1,118
AIDS[b]	1,501	1,607	1,731
Minority AIDS	282	300	323
Pediatric AIDS	165	174	188
Vaccines	130	153	180
Alzheimer's disease	329	349	375
Biotechnology research	5,147	5,453	5,898
Cancer research[a]	2,761	2,942	3,232
Breast cancer[a]	411	433	458
Breast cancer, genetic	95	100	106
Lung cancer	143	151	161
Prostate cancer	105	114	122
Cardiovascular research	1,080	1,155	1,223
Chronic fatigue syndrome	7	8	8
Cystic fibrosis	70	74	79
Decade of the brain (brain disorders)	2,539	2,696	2,902
Diabetes[c]	320	373	415
Diagnostic radiology	239	249	269
Diethylstilbestrol	4	5	5
Emerging infectious diseases	90	99	108
Epstein-Barr virus	24	25	27
Chronic fatigue syndrome	7	8	8
Fibromyalgia	2	3	3
Gene mapping	848	915	988
Gene therapy	253	269	288
Health and behavioral research	904	954	1,027
Hepatitis C	25	30	34
Human fetal tissue research	19	20	21
Hypertension	165	175	189
Immunology	1,274	1,357	1,458
Infant mortality (low birth weight)	314	331	353
Kidney disease	196	209	225
Lupus	34	36	39
Nutrition	452	474	507
Osteoporosis[a]	112	121	132

Continued

TABLE C-4 *Continued*

Disease or Area of Research	FY 1997 Budget Authority	FY 1998 Estimate	FY 1999 Estimate
Parkinson's disease	$89	$98	$107
Direct	36	41	45
Indirect	54	57	62
Pediatric research	1,604	1,706	1,837
Prevention[a]	3,225	3,455	3,751
NCI primary prevention	486	510	528
Rehabilitation	171	182	196
Rural health	98	102	109
Schizophrenia	111	117	126
Sexually transmitted diseases/herpes	120	128	138
Sickle cell disease	49	53	57
Sleep disorders	85	88	95
Smoking and health	287	307	333
Spinal cord injury	61	65	70
Stroke[a]	143	152	165
Sudden infant death syndrome	44	47	50
Topical microbicides	20	23	26
Tobacco research	420	449	486
Tropical diseases	114	122	132
Tuberculosis research	67	69	70
Vaccine development	298	337	377
Vaccine-related research	336	377	418
Women's health research[a]	1,978	2,110	2,278
Youth and tobacco	32	36	42

NOTE: Data do not reflect funds for breast cancer research associated with the FY 1997 Budget Supplement ($15 million).

[a]Reflects the effect of the Women's Health Initiative transfer in all years.
[b]Represents budget authority for AIDS.
[c]Includes transfer of $27 million for type I diabetes research for FY 1998–2002 in accordance with the Balanced Budget Act.

SOURCE: Office of Financial Management, NIH, 1998.

TABLE C-5 NIH Funding from the Cancer Research Initiative by Institute, Center, and Division (in thousands of dollars)

Institute, Center, or Division	FY 1997 Estimate	FY 1998 Estimate	FY 1999 Estimate
NCI	$2,389,041	$2,547,314	$2,776,267
NHLBI[a]	57,620	59,815	67,539
NIDR	16,448	17,313	19,811
NIDDK	33,430	36,450	39,350
NINDS	17,929	18,734	24,468
NIAID	43,085	44,377	47,927
NIGMS	22,574	24,421	30,421
NICHD	10,311	11,000	11,900
NEI	8,616	9,242	9,508
NIEHS	84,368	89,430	94,796
NIA	12,183	12,730	14,990
NIAMS	5,303	5,690	6,220
NIDCD	2,910	3,087	4,296
NIMH	3,720	3,823	4,116
NIDA	0	0	0
NIAAA	1,717	2,000	2,500
NINR	3,978	4,250	4,570
NHGRI	20,758	22,158	30,151
NCRR	26,162	28,754	37,874
FIC	545	575	600
NLM	0	0	4,500
Total budget authority	2,760,698	2,941,163	3,231,804

[a]Reflects the effect of the Women's Health Initiative transfer in all years.

SOURCE: Office of Financial Management, NIH, 1998.

TABLE C-6 NIH Funding from the Diabetes Research Initiative by Institute, Center, and Division (in thousands of dollars)

Institute, Center, or Division	FY 1997 Estimate	FY 1998 Estimate	FY 1999 Estimate
NCI	$1,164	$1,000	$1,029
NHLBI	21,270	22,744	28,504
NIDR	2,807	2,956	3,042
NIDDK	211,626	229,000	256,641
NINDS	3,461	4,076	4,194
NIAID	9,231	9,117	9,381
NIGMS	—	—	2,000
NICHD	16,042	17,100	17,596
NEI	21,604	23,172	25,844
NIEHS	517	1,317	1,355
NIA	6,416	8,190	8,428
NIMH	1,462	1,840	1,893
NIAAA	1,069	1,110	1,142
NINR	705	750	772
NHGRI	2,704	2,895	4479
NCRR	19,461	20,784	21,387
FIC	—	164	169
Total budget authority	319,539	373,215	414,856

NOTE: Total budget authority includes transfer of $27 million for type I diabetes research in accordance with the Balanced Budget Act.

SOURCE: Office of Financial Management, NIH, 1998.

TABLE C-7 Estimates of Costs and NIH Support of Related Research for the 10 Leading Diseases or Conditions Causing Death in the United States

Disease or Condition	No. of Deaths (in thousands; 1994)	Cost Estimate (in $ billions)		NIH Support in FY 1996 (in $ millions)
		Direct	Indirect[a]	
Heart diseases	732.4	$70.9[b]	$54.9	$851.6
Cancer	534.3	27.5[c]	68.7	2,570.6
Stroke	153.3	17.0[d]	13.0	120.3
Chronic obstructive pulmonary disease and allied conditions	101.6	16.5[b]	11.1	62.4
Pneumonia and influenza	81.5	18.2[b]	3.9	61.9
Diabetes	56.7	45.2[e]	46.6	298.9
HIV infection and AIDS	42.1	10.3[e]	NA	1,410.9
Chronic liver disease and cirrhosis	25.4	1.2[f]	2.1	169.8
Kidney and urologic diseases	23.0	26.2[f]	14.1	327.2
Septicemia	20.4	4.2[b]	NA	10.9

NOTE: This list excludes non-disease-related causes of death: homicide, suicide, and injury. FY = fiscal year; NA = not available; and HIV = human immunodeficiency virus.

[a]Indirect costs include costs due to mortality of patient (premature death), morbidity of patient (reduced productivity), services of unpaid caregivers, and other related non-health-care costs.
[b]Year of reference, 1991.
[c]Year of reference, 1990.
[d]Year of reference, 1993.
[e]Year of reference, 1992.
[f]Year of reference, 1985.

SOURCE: National Institutes of Health, 1997a.

D

Committee and Staff Biographies

COMMITTEE BIOGRAPHIES

LEON E. ROSENBERG, M.D., is a Professor in the Department of Molecular Biology and the Woodrow Wilson School of Public and International Affairs at Princeton University. He formerly served at Bristol-Myers Squibb Company as President of the Pharmaceutical Research Institute and as Senior Vice President of Scientific Affairs. Prior to joining Bristol-Myers Squibb, Dr. Rosenberg was Dean of the Yale University School of Medicine. During his 26-year affiliation with Yale, Dr. Rosenberg worked as a research geneticist, teacher, clinician, and administrator. Dr. Rosenberg received B.A. and M.D. degrees, both summa cum laude, from the University of Wisconsin. He completed his internship and residency training in internal medicine at Columbia-Presbyterian Medical Center in New York City. Active in professional societies, Dr. Rosenberg is a fellow of the American Academy of Arts and Sciences and the American Association for the Advancement of Science. He is a past president of the American Society of Human Genetics and of the Association of American Physicians. Dr. Rosenberg is a member of the National Academy of Sciences and the Institute of Medicine.

JOHN F. ALDERETE, Ph.D., is Professor of Microbiology at the University of Texas Health Science Center at San Antonio. His undergraduate B.S. degrees in both mathematics and biology were from the New Mexico Institute of Mining and Technology at Socorro. Dr. Alderete received a Ph.D. in microbiology from the University of Kansas, Lawrence. He has published close to 100 publications in peer-reviewed journals and is the author of 15 book chapters. Dr. Alderete has been a member of numerous study sections and panels for several of the institutes at the National Institutes of Health, the National Science Foundation, and other government agencies. He is a member of the board of the Intercultural

Cancer Council. He is often asked to speak to students, parent groups, and organizations across the country on issues involving minorities and higher education and on American workforce issues. These groups and organizations include the President's National Science Board, the National Institutes of Health, the U.S. Food and Drug Administration, and, more recently, the President's Office of Science and Technology Policy. Dr. Alderete is the President of the Society for the Advancement of Chicanos and Native Americans in the Sciences, one of the fastest-growing and highest-quality minority science societies in the United States.

KENNETH B. CHANCE, D.D.S., is Dean and Professor of Endodontics at the School of Dentistry at Meharry Medical College. Dr. Chance graduated with a bachelor of science degree in biology from Fordham University. He earned a doctor of dental surgery degree from Case Western Reserve University in 1979. Dr. Chance also completed a general dentistry residency at Jamaica Hospital in New York City and holds a certificate in endodontics from the University of Medicine and Dentistry of New Jersey (UMDNJ), New Jersey Dental School. Dr. Chance's academic and administrative appointments have included Associate Professor, UMDNJ, New Jersey Dental School; Chief of Endodontics, Kings County Medical Center, Brooklyn, N.Y.; and Director, Health Policy Program of the Joint Center for Political and Economic Studies, Washington, D.C. He is the recipient of several honors and awards. He was a Robert Wood Johnson Health Policy and Pew National Leadership Fellow from 1991 to 1992. Dr. Chance is a fellow of the American and International College of Dentists and the Pierre Fauchard Academy.

CARON CHESS, Ph.D., is Director of Rutgers University's Center for Environmental Communication, which conducts research and training to improve communication about environmental issues. Her experience in academia, government, and environmental advocacy underpins her research interests and publications. Dr. Chess has coauthored publications that are used widely by government and industry practitioners. Her current research interests include methods of evaluating public participation and study of the impact of organizational factors on public participation and risk communication. Dr. Chess received a B.A. degree in English from the State University of New York at Buffalo, an M.S. degree in environmental communications from the University of Michigan, and a Ph.D. degree in environmental studies and democratic processes from the State University of New York. Dr. Chess has served on the Committee on Risk Characterization and Board on Radioactive Waste Management of the National Academy of Sciences. She also has been a member of the governing board of the Society for Risk Analysis.

PURNELL CHOPPIN, M.D., is President of the Howard Hughes Medical Institute. Dr. Choppin was Leon Hess Professor of Virology, Vice President for Academic Programs, Dean of Graduate Studies, and Head of the Laboratory of Virology at the Rockefeller University. Before joining The Rockefeller University as a fellow and as a faculty member, he served as an intern and resident in internal medicine at the Washington University School of Medicine and Barnes Hospital in St. Louis and as a medical officer in the Air Force. He received a medical degree from the Louisiana State University School of Medicine. Dr. Choppin is a past chairman of Class IV (medical sciences) and of the Section on Microbiology and Immunology of the National Academy of Sciences. He has served as a member of the Council and Executive Committee of the Institute of Medicine and as a member of the Governing Board of the National Research Council. He received the Selman A. Waksman Award for excellence in microbiology from the National Academy of Sciences. Dr. Choppin is a member of the National Academy of Sciences and the Institute of Medicine.

JAMES W. CURRAN, M.D., Ph.D., is Professor of Epidemiology and Dean of the Rollins School of Public Health of Emory University. He serves as Director of the Emory/Atlanta Center for AIDS Research. Dr. Curran graduated from the University of Notre Dame with a bachelor of science degree. He received a medical degree from the University of Michigan and a master of public health degree from the Harvard University School of Public Health. Dr. Curran was a fellow at the Harvard Center for Community Health and Medical Care. Dr. Curran began his career with the Centers for Disease Control and Prevention, where he held leadership positions in AIDS research and prevention activities until 1995. Dr. Curran is a member of the Institute of Medicine.

DAVID M. CUTLER, Ph.D., is Professor of Economics at Harvard University, in the Economics Department, and at the Kennedy School of Government. Dr. Cutler is also a Research Associate at the National Bureau of Economic Research. He received a B.A., summa cum laude, from Harvard College and a Ph.D. in economics from the Massachusetts Institute of Technology. Dr. Cutler's research is concentrated in health economics, including explanations for increasing health costs, the effect of managed care on medical outcomes, and measuring the productivity of the medical sector. Dr. Cutler was recently named Editor of the *Journal of Health Economics*. During 1993, Dr. Cutler was on leave as Senior Staff Economist at the Council of Economic Advisers and Director of the National Economic Council in the Clinton Administration. Dr. Cutler's primary responsibilities were in helping to design the president's health reform plan.

SUE K. DONALDSON, Ph.D., R.N., is Professor and Dean of the School of Nursing and Professor of Physiology, School of Medicine at Johns Hopkins

University. She received B.S.N. and M.S.N. degrees from Wayne State University and a Ph.D. in physiology and biophysics from the University of Washington. Before coming to Johns Hopkins, Dr. Donaldson was Professor of Physiology, School of Medicine, as well as Professor, Cora Meidl Siehl Endowed Research Chair, and Director of the Center for Long-Term Care of the Elderly, School of Nursing, University of Minnesota. Dr. Donaldson is a pioneer in nursing research and is internationally known for her basic science research in cellular skeletal and cardiac muscle physiology. In 1992, Dr. Donaldson was inducted as a fellow in the American Academy of Nursing. Dr. Donaldson is a member of the Institute of Medicine.

BARUCH FISCHHOFF, Ph.D., is University Professor of Social and Decision Sciences and of Engineering and Public Policy at Carnegie Mellon University. He holds a B.S. in mathematics from Wayne State University and an M.A. and a Ph.D. in psychology from the Hebrew University of Jerusalem. He is a fellow of the American Psychological Association and a recipient of its Early Career Awards for Distinguished Scientific Contribution to Psychology and for Contributions to Psychology in the Public Interest. He is a fellow of the Society for Risk Analysis, as well as recipient of its Distinguished Achievement Award. Dr. Fischhoff's areas of research include risk communication, risk management, adolescent decision making, evaluation of environmental damages, and protective behavior. He serves on the editorial boards of several journals. He is a member of the Institute of Medicine.

SID GILMAN, M.D., is the William J. Herdman Professor and Chair of the Department of Neurology at the University of Michigan and Chief of the Neurology Service at the University of Michigan Hospitals. He also serves as Director of the Michigan Alzheimer's Disease Research Center. Dr. Gilman received his undergraduate and medical training at the University of California, Los Angeles (UCLA). After his internship in internal medicine at the UCLA Hospital, he served as a research associate at the National Institutes of Health for 2 years and then as a resident in neurology at the Harvard Medical School/Boston City Hospital. After serving as a fellow, he became a faculty member at Harvard Medical School. He then moved to the College of Physicians and Surgeons of Columbia University, where he rose through the ranks quickly and became the H. Houston Merritt Professor of Neurology. He assumed his present position in 1977. Dr. Gilman's research involves both basic science and clinical investigations focused upon neurodegenerative diseases, including Parkinson's disease, cerebellar degeneration, and Alzheimer's disease. He currently serves as Chair of the Peripheral and Central Nervous System Drugs Advisory Committee of the U.S. Food and Drug Administration. Dr. Gilman has received many prestigious awards and honors. He has served as President of the American Neurological

Association and of the Michigan Neurological Association. Dr. Gilman is a member of the Institute of Medicine.

ROBERT L. HILL, Ph.D., is the James B. Duke Professor of the Department of Biochemistry at Duke University Medical Center. He has trained more than 100 Ph.D. students and postdoctoral fellows while at Duke University. Dr. Hill has served as President of the American Society of Biochemistry and Molecular Biology (ASBMB) and was chair of the Organizing Committee of the Joint Meeting of the 17th International Congress of ASBMB. He has been a consultant to the National Institutes of Health for review of research grants and training grants and has served on the Director's Advisory Committee. Dr. Hill received an A.B., an M.A., and a Ph.D. from the University of Kansas. He is Associate Editor of the *Journal of Biological Chemistry*. Dr. Hill is a member of the National Academy of Sciences and the Institute of Medicine.

RALPH I. HORWITZ, M.D., is Harold H. Hines, Jr., Professor of Medicine and Epidemiology and Chairman of the Department of Internal Medicine at the Yale University School of Medicine and Codirector of the Yale Robert Wood Johnson Clinical Scholars Program. Dr. Horwitz's scientific interests are in clinical research and epidemiology and emphasize especially methodologies for studying the strategies of clinical care. His prior Institute of Medicine committee memberships include the Committee on Persian Gulf Syndrome Comprehensive Clinical Evaluation Program and the Committee on Policies for Allocating Health Sciences Research Funds. Dr. Horwitz is a member of the Institute of Medicine.

THOMAS KELLY, M.D., Ph.D., is the Boury Professor and Chairman of the Department of Molecular Biology and Genetics at the Johns Hopkins University School of Medicine. His scientific interests are in the enzymology and regulation of DNA replication in eukaryotic cells. He received B.A., M.D., and Ph.D. degrees from the Johns Hopkins University and was a postdoctoral fellow at Harvard Medical School and the Johns Hopkins University School of Medicine. He served for 2 years in the U.S. Public Health Service as a Staff Associate at the National Institutes of Health. Dr. Kelly has been a frequent consultant to the National Institutes of Health for review of research grants and was a member of the Panel to Assess the NIH Investment in Gene Therapy. He also serves as a member of the National Cancer Policy Board. Dr. Kelly is a fellow of the American Philosophical Society and the American Academy of Arts and Sciences and a member of the National Academy of Sciences.

ANNE C. PETERSEN, Ph.D., is Senior Vice President for Programs at the W. K. Kellogg Foundation. Dr. Petersen oversees the development of effective programming strategies, fosters teamwork, and develops and monitors policies, philosophies, and organization-wide systems for accomplishing the programmatic mission of the foundation. Previously, Dr. Petersen was the Deputy Director of the National Science Foundation. She was the first woman in the agency's 45-year history to serve in that position. She also served as the Vice President for Research and Dean of the Graduate School at the University of Minnesota. Dr. Petersen has authored many books and articles on adolescence, gender, and research methods. Dr. Petersen holds a bachelor's degree in mathematics, a master's degree in statistics, and a doctorate in measurement, evaluation, and statistical analysis, all from the University of Chicago.

SUSAN C. SCRIMSHAW, Ph.D., is Dean, School of Public Health, and Professor of Community Health Sciences and Anthropology, University of Illinois-Chicago. She was a Professor of Public Health and Anthropology at the University of California, Los Angeles (UCLA), and Associate Dean for Academic Programs for the School of Public Health of UCLA. She is an anthropologist who is especially tuned to Hispanic and African-American public health issues. Dr. Scrimshaw's research interests are cross-cultural work on health access, health behavior, improving pregnancy outcomes, rapid anthropological assessment, combining qualitative and quantitative methods, Latino culture in the United States and Latin America, women's health, AIDS, and managing cultural diversity. She is a fellow of the American Association for the Advancement of Science and has received numerous awards for her work, including the 1985 Margaret Mead Award from the Society for Applied Anthropology and the American Anthropological Association. She has served on many National Academy of Sciences and Institute of Medicine panels and committees, most recently, the Board on International Health. Dr. Scrimshaw is a member of the Institute of Medicine.

ROGER H. UNGER, M.D., is Professor of Internal Medicine at the Center for Diabetes Research at the University of Texas Southwestern Medical Center. Dr. Unger has received the Banting Medal of the American Diabetes Association, the Rumbaugh Award of the Juvenile Diabetes Foundation, the Koch Award of the Endocrine Society, the Claude Bernard Medal of the European Associates for the Study of Diabetes, and a Senior Medical Investigatorship of the Veterans Affairs Medical Center in Dallas, Texas. Dr. Unger has been Director of the Center for Diabetes Research since 1986. He is Professor of Internal Medicine and the Touchstone/West Distinguished Chair in Diabetes Research. Dr. Unger is a member of the American Academy of Arts and Sciences, as well as a member of the National Academy of Sciences.

MYRL WEINBERG, CAE, is President of the National Health Council, an umbrella organization encompassing more than 100 national health-related groups. Previously, Ms. Weinberg served as Vice President for Corporate

Relations and Public Affairs for the American Diabetes Association (ADA) and was in charge of government relations, public relations, and corporate marketing. Prior to that, she served for 5 years as ADA's Vice President for Programs and the group's first Director of Government Relations. Prior to joining ADA, Ms. Weinberg was Director of Program Development for the Joseph P. Kennedy, Jr., Foundation and earlier worked as Assistant Director of Government Relations for ARC (formerly the Association for Retarded Citizens). Ms. Weinberg has a long history of board and committee service, including work with the National Chronic Care Consortium's National Resource Center, the American Medical Association's Ethical FORCE initiative, the American Society of Association Executives' Ethics Committee, the Funding First Program, the Foundation for Accountability, the National Legal Center for the Medically Dependent and Disabled, Inc., and the Accreditation for Services for Mentally Retarded and Other Developmentally Disabled Persons. She holds an M.A. in special education from George Peabody College and a B.A. in psychology from the University of Arkansas.

LINDA S. WILSON, Ph.D., is President of Radcliffe College. She served as Vice President for Research at the University of Michigan. A graduate of Sophie Newcomb College, Tulane University, Dr. Wilson earned a Ph.D. in inorganic chemistry at the University of Wisconsin. Dr. Wilson now leads an educational institution devoted to the advancement of society through the advancement of women through education, research, and public policy. She is noted particularly for her efforts to develop cooperative working relationships among universities, government, and industry and for her attention to individual, institutional, and systemic issues in the development of science and engineering personnel. Her publications span the fields of chemistry, science policy, higher education, and women's education. Dr. Wilson is a fellow of the American Association for the Advancement of Science. Dr. Wilson is a member of the Institute of Medicine.

ADAM YARMOLINSKY, LL.B., is the Regent's Professor of Public Policy in the University of Maryland system. He was Provost and Professor in the Graduate Program in Policy Sciences at the University of Maryland Baltimore County campus from 1985 to 1993. He served in the Kennedy, Johnson, and Carter administrations in the White House, the Pentagon, and the Arms Control and Disarmament Agency. Mr. Yarmolinsky is a founding member of the Institute of Medicine.

STAFF BIOGRAPHIES

ANDREW M. POPE, Ph.D., is the Director of the Health Sciences Policy Program at the Institute of Medicine. With expertise in physiology, toxicology, and epidemiology, his primary interests focus on environmental and occupational influences on human health. As a research fellow in the Division of Pharmacology and Toxicology at the U.S. Food and Drug Administration, Dr. Pope's research focused on the biochemical, neuroendocrine, and reproductive effects of various environmental substances on food-producing animals. During his tenure at the National Academy of Sciences and since 1989 at the Institute of Medicine, Dr. Pope has directed and edited numerous reports on environmental and occupational issues; topics include injury control, disability prevention, biologic markers, neurotoxicology, indoor allergens, and the inclusion of environmental and occupational health content in medical and nursing school curricula.

GEOFFREY S. FRENCH is a Research Associate in the Health Sciences Policy Program. He has been with the Institute of Medicine (IOM) for 3 years, having supported the Office of Finance and Administration and the IOM committees that produced the reports *Enabling America: Assessing the Role of Rehabilitation Science and Engineering* and *Halcion: An Independent Assessment of Safety and Efficacy Data.* His undergraduate degree is in history and anthropology, and he completed his master's degree in national security studies at Georgetown University.

CHARLES H. EVANS, JR., M.D., Ph.D., is the Head of the Health Sciences Section in the Institute of Medicine. Dr. Evans joined the staff of the Institute of Medicine in March 1998. As Head of the new Health Sciences Section, Dr. Evans has management responsibility for all scientific, administrative, and financial affairs of the Health Sciences Section, which includes the Health Sciences Policy Program and the Neuroscience and Behavioral Health Program and their respective boards in the Institute of Medicine. Dr. Evans is a pediatrician and immunologist and holds the rank of Captain (retired) in the U.S. Public Health Service with 27 years of service as a medical scientist at the National Institutes of Health. He received his B.S. (biology) degree from Union College in 1962 and M.D. and Ph.D. (microbiology) degrees from the University of Virginia in 1969. He was an intern and resident in pediatrics at the University of Virginia from 1969 to 1971 and from 1971 to 1998 served as a Medical Officer in the U.S. Public Health Service Commissioned Corps and concurrently from 1976 to 1998 was Chief of the Tumor Biology Section at the National Cancer Institute. An expert in carcinogenesis and the normal immune system defenses to the development of cancer, he is the author of more than 250 scientific publications. He and his laboratory colleagues discovered the cytokine leukoregulin in 1983 and were awarded three U.S. patents. Dr. Evans has been active as an adviser to community medicine and higher education through his service on the Board of Trustees of Suburban Hospital Health System (1988 to present) and on the Arts and Sciences Alumni Council at the University of Virginia (1987 to 1997). He is the recipient of numerous scientific awards including the Outstanding Service Medal from the U.S. Public Health Service and the Wellcome Medal and Prize. Dr. Evans has been a member of the editorial boards of several scientific journals, has served on a variety of scientific advisory committees, and is a Fellow of the American Institute of Chemists and a credentialed Fellow in Health Systems Administration of the American Academy of Medical Administrators.

ROBERT M. COOK-DEEGAN, M.D., directs the National Cancer Policy Board of the Institute of Medicine (IOM) and Commission on Life Sciences, National Academy of Sciences. He previously worked as staff for the report *Allocating Federal Funds for Science and Technology* (the Press Report) for the National Academy of Sciences and directed an IOM division (now Neuroscience and Behavioral Health Program). He was acting executive director of the congressional Biomedical Ethics Advisory Committee in 1989 following 6 years at the Office of Technology Assessment. He is the author of *The Gene Wars: Science, Politics, and the Human Genome*. He chairs the Royalty Fund Advisory Committee for the Alzheimer's Association, was a founding member of the Dana Alliance for Brain Initiatives, and is retiring chair of Section X (Social Impacts of Science and Engineering) for the American Association for the Advancement of Science.

KATHI E. HANNA, Ph.D., is a science and health policy consultant specializing in biomedical research policy, specifically, genetics, cancer, and reproductive technologies. Most recently, Dr. Hanna served as Senior Advisor to the National Bioethics Advisory Commission in its response to the president's request for recommendations regarding human cloning. Prior to that she was Senior Advisor to the President's Advisory Committee on Gulf War Veterans Illnesses, in which she assessed the effects of military service on the reproductive health of veterans. Dr. Hanna was a senior analyst at the congressional Office of Technology Assessment for 7 years and contributed to numerous science policy studies requested by committees of the U.S. Congress on biotechnology, human genetics, women's health, reproductive technologies, and bioethics. In 1989, Dr. Hanna spent a year at the Institute of Medicine where she edited a book about the interface between biomedical research and politics. In the past decade, Dr. Hanna has also served as a consultant to the Howard Hughes Medical Institute, the National Institutes of Health, the Institute of Medicine, the Federation of American Societies of Experimental Biology, and several academic health centers. Prior to her work in Washington, D.C., Dr. Hanna was the Genetics Coordinator at Children's Memorial Hospital in Chicago. Dr. Hanna received an A.B. in biology from Lafayette College, an M.S. in human genetics from Sarah Lawrence College, and a doctorate from the School of Business and Public Management, George Washington University.

MICHAEL McGEARY is a political scientist who directed the staff work for a dozen reports by committees of the Institute of Medicine (IOM) and other units of the National Academy of Sciences (NAS) between 1981 and 1995, including reports on the cancer centers program of the National Cancer Institute and the AIDS research program of the National Institutes of Health. He did his graduate work at the Massachusetts Institute of Technology and, prior to going to NAS, taught at Wellesley College and worked at the National Academy of Public Administration. Currently, he is a consultant on federal science and technology policy, funding, and organization and is coauthoring a book on U.S. science and technology policy. He has served as a consultant to IOM, the National Research Council (Office of Scientific and Engineering Personnel), NAS (Committee on Science, Engineering, and Public Policy), the Association of American Universities, SRI International, Alzheimer's Association, and Washington Advisory Group.